AN INTRODUCTION TO
THE BIOLOGY OF VISION

AN INTRODUCTION TO
THE BIOLOGY OF VISION

JAMES T. McILWAIN
Brown University

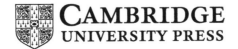

CAMBRIDGE UNIVERSITY PRESS
Cambridge, New York, Melbourne, Madrid, Cape Town, Singapore, São Paulo

Cambridge University Press
The Edinburgh Building, Cambridge CB2 2RU, UK

Published in the United States of America by Cambridge University Press, New York

www.cambridge.org
Information on this title: www.cambridge.org/9780521495486

First published 1996
Reprinted 1998

A catalogue record for this publication is available from the British Library

ISBN-13 978-0-521-49548-6 hardback
ISBN-10 0-521-49548-2 hardback

ISBN-13 978-0-521-49890-6 paperback
ISBN-10 0-521-49890-2 paperback

Transferred to digital printing 2006

To my teachers

CONTENTS

PREFACE

This textbook is an attempt to answer a question: What would I want a student to know about the visual system before beginning work in my laboratory? Draft versions have been used for several years in an undergraduate course at Brown University. Inevitably, the content and approach of the book have been colored by my expectations of students in that course and by my own particular interests. It is assumed that students will have had an introductory course on the nervous system and will be acquainted with the fundamentals of cellular neurophysiology and the general organization of the vertebrate central nervous system. Minimal knowledge of physics is assumed, so some time will be spent on the elementary principles of optics as they apply to visual systems. Although the book is intended primarily for undergraduates, it can provide useful background for beginning graduate students if supplemented by material from the research literature.

The text is organized into three parts. Part I treats the eye as an image-forming organ and provides an overview of the projections from the retina to key visual structures of the brain. Part II examines the functions of the retina and its central projections in greater detail, building on the introductory material of Part I. Part III treats certain special topics in vision that require this detailed knowledge of the structure and properties of the retina and visual projections. Each chapter ends with a list of additional readings selected principally from reviews and monographs. These will provide access to the primary literature for the student who wishes to pursue a subject in greater depth.

The emphasis here is on the vertebrate visual system, although examples from the invertebrate world are introduced whenever contrast and comparison are instructive. This bias flows from the conviction that most undergraduate college students are interested primarily in their own brains and visual systems and that the riches of the invertebrate world seem remote and exotic. Because invertebrate approaches to the exploitation of light are in many ways more interesting than the vertebrate pattern, it is hoped that some students, at least, will be stimulated to pursue a more systematic study of invertebrate vision.

I have benefited greatly from comments on various chapters offered by Vivien Casagrande, Michael Rowe, Leslie Welch, Billy Wooten, and Anita Zimmerman. Katherine Fite read the entire manuscript and contributed valuable suggestions on content and presentation. Ellen Grass, AstroMed Inc., and Trudy Nicholson, the artist, graciously gave permission to use the drawing of a bush baby that appears on the cover. Errors and omissions remain the responsibility of the author, as he will doubtless be reminded.

PART I

THE EYE AND VISUAL PATHWAYS

CHAPTER 1

INTRODUCTION

The physicist Richard Feynman once illustrated the extraordinary nature of vision as follows: We are immersed in a sea of electromagnetic waves whose lengths vary over a huge range (Figure 1.1). These waves interact with each other and with objects around us to present a cacophony of electromagnetic signals to our eyes. Through a tiny aperture, about 2 mm in diameter, the eye selects a small fraction of these wavelengths and, together with the brain, reconstructs the position, shape, color, and motion of each object we see around us. Feynman compared the situation to that of a water bug floating on the surface at one corner of a swimming pool. The only information available to the bug comes from the movements of its body caused by the waves that reach it. Were the bug able to reconstruct from these waves the positions and motions of all the people entering, leaving, and swimming in the pool, it would be doing something similar to what the eye and brain do with the minuscule electromagnetic disturbances passing through the pupil.

Why does the eye normally respond only to electromagnetic energy with wavelengths in the range 400–700 nm (1 nm = 10^{-9} m)? To answer this question, one must ask what electromagnetic energy was available to the earliest living forms that developed vision. The major source of such energy reaching the surface of the earth is the sun, which emits radiation with the spectrum shown in Figure 1.2. Note that the energy peaks near 500 nm, within the visual range, but it also extends to longer and shorter

3

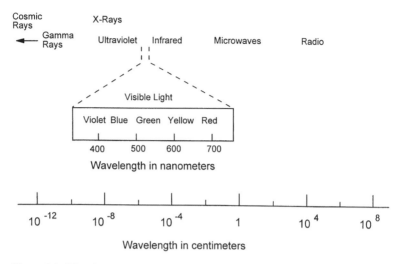

Visible Light

Violet Blue Green Yellow Red

| 400 | 500 | 600 | 700 |

Wavelength in nanometers

10 ⁻¹²   10 ⁻⁸   10 ⁻⁴   1   10 ⁴   10 ⁸

Wavelength in centimeters

Figure 1.1. The electromagnetic spectrum.

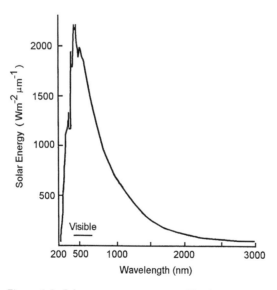

Figure 1.2. Solar-energy spectrum outside the atmosphere. (Reprinted, with permission, from D. M. Gates: Spectral distribution of solar radiation at the earth's surface. *Science* 151:523–8. Copyright 1966, American Association for the Advancement of Science.)

wavelengths. As this solar radiation passes through the atmosphere, the intensity of ultraviolet rays is reduced by the ozone layer, and that of infrared rays by water vapor, narrowing the effective range of wavelengths reaching the earth's surface. Further filtering occurs in sea water, which exhibits a window of minimal attenuation at those wavelengths we call light.

Figure 1.3 compares the spectral content of light above and below the ocean's surface with the spectral sensitivities of the rod and cone systems of human vision. (Differences between the two types of photoreceptors subserving these systems will be discussed later.) Our eyes, like those of many other animals, detect that narrow range of wavelengths available beneath the surface of the sea, where the earliest visual systems emerged. Some animals, such as certain species of birds and insects, can see ultraviolet light, but even this sensitivity is restricted to the so-called near-ultraviolet, wavelengths not much shorter than those sensed by our own eyes. Pit vipers can sense infrared radiation, but they do this with specialized somatic sensory receptors, not with their eyes.

In order to use the energy available from the sun, the earliest living organisms required molecules with very special properties. First, these molecules had to absorb the available electromagnetic energy without being destroyed, and then they had to divert the energy in some way to useful biological processes. Several molecules emerged to accomplish this, perhaps the most important of which is chlorophyll. Virtually all living creatures depend directly or indirectly on the ability of chlorophyll-containing cells to synthesize carbohydrates from carbon dioxide and water and release oxygen into the environment. In fact, the development of the ozone layer required the evolution of photosynthesis in microorganisms of the sea, a process that made terrestrial life possible by shielding nucleic acids and other vital cellular elements from destructive ultraviolet radiation.

Phototropism in plants and vision in animals depend largely on another group of compounds, the carotenoids. A special class of these, the retinoids, play important roles in development and cell metabolism through actions that are still imperfectly understood. They may act as cofactors in important biochemical reactions and may also regulate gene expression. One of these retinoids, the 11-*cis* isomer of retinal, is the aldehyde of vitamin A and has the important property of changing shape when it absorbs light within the band of wavelengths available from the sun. The visual photopigments in all multicellular animals are formed by combining 11-*cis* retinal, the chromophore, with a large, membrane-bound protein called an opsin. The opsins of visual photopigments are members of a large family of membrane-spanning molecules, most of which sense chemical stimuli outside the cell and regulate critical biochemical processes within the cell.

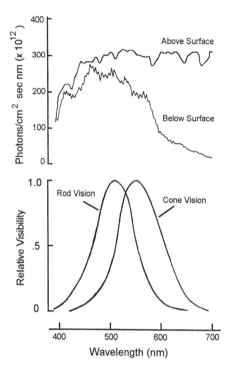

Figure 1.3. Top panel: Comparison of solar spectra measured just above and 3 m below the surface of the clear tropical sea at Eniwetok. (Reprinted from W. N. McFarland and F. W. Munz: The photic environment of clear tropical seas during the day. *Vision Research* 15:1063–70. Copyright 1975, with kind permission from Elsevier Science, Ltd., The Boulevard, Langford Lane, Kidlington OX5 1GB, United Kingdom.) Bottom panel: Spectral sensitivities of human rod and cone vision. (Reprinted from S. Hecht and R. E. Williams: The visibility of mono-chromatic radiation and the absorption spectrum of visual purple. *Journal of General Physiology* 5:1–34. Copyright 1922, with permission of the Rockefeller University Press.)

Figure 1.4 illustrates schematically the family resemblance of some of the better known of these membrane receptors.

Just as the cow's opsin of Figure 1.4 is related structurally to various membrane receptors of humans, hamsters, turkeys, and pigs, the photo-pigment opsins of various species bear striking similarities in their amino acid sequences, indicating that they are derived from an ancient common ancestor. The diagram of Figure 1.5 illustrates schematically the resem-blances among several opsins from species as evolutionarily divergent as fruit flies and humans: The greater the sequence similarity of any two opsins, the shorter the distances along the line segments connecting them.

Cytoplasmic Space

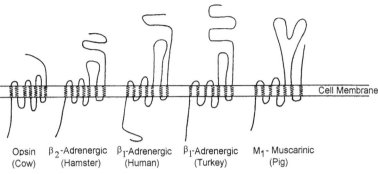

Opsin	β_2-Adrenergic	β_1-Adrenergic	β_1-Adrenergic	M_1- Muscarinic
(Cow)	(Hamster)	(Human)	(Turkey)	(Pig)

Extracellular Space

Figure 1.4. Examples from a family of membrane-spanning proteins serving photoreception (far left) and receptors for adrenergic and muscarinic cholinergic neurotransmitters. All have seven transmembrane segments, but their intracellular and extracellular domains differ in length. (Adapted from E. R. Weiss, D. J. Kelleher, C. W. Woon, S. Soparkar, S. Osawa, L. E. Heasley, and G. L. Johnson: Receptor activation of G proteins. *FASEB Journal* 2:2841–8, 1994, with permission of the Federation of American Societies for Experimental Biology.)

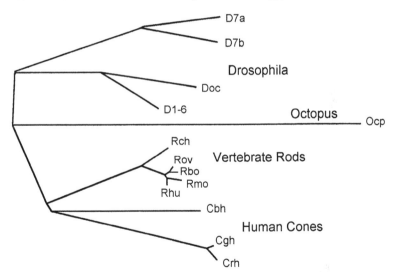

Figure 1.5. Evolutionary distances between various opsins. The distance along a line connecting two opsins reflects the difference in their amino acid compositions. D, *Drosophila* rhodopsins; Ocp, octopus rhodopsin. Vertebrate rod opsins: Rch, chicken; Rbo, cow; Rov, sheep; Rmo, mouse; Rhu, human. Human cone opsins: Cbh, Cgh, and Crh are human short-, medium-, and long-wavelength cones, respectively. (Adapted from T. H. Goldsmith: Optimization, constraint, and history in the evolution of eyes. *Quarterly Review of Biology* 65:281–322, 1990, with permission of The University of Chicago Press.)

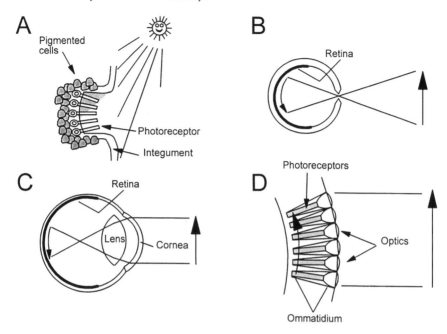

Figure 1.6. Varieties of eyes. (A) An eye spot, such as that found in *Planaria*. (B) An eye that uses a pin-hole aperture to form images. Such an eye occurs in *Nautilus*. (C) Vertebrate-type camera eye using a lens and cornea for image formation. (D) Compound eye, such as that of the horseshoe crab, *Limulus polyphemus*.

Even though the photopigments of all animals share a common ancestor, this is not true of their eyes. Vertebrate and invertebrate eyes differ in many important ways, and no definite ancestral link has been established between them. The same can be said for various forms of eyes among invertebrates. The most primitive eyes probably were clusters of photosensitive cells gathered together in pigmented pits called eye spots (Figure 1.6A). Eye spots serve to signal relative degrees of light and darkness and appear to have evolved independently many times. The pigmented cells lining the pit bestow some directional sensitivity on the eye spot by preventing light from reaching the photoreceptors through the often transparent bodies of the small invertebrate animals. If the pits are deep enough, shadows cast by the walls of the pit on different parts of the receptor array provide additional directional information, which can serve an animal well when it needs to escape at the sudden appearance of a predator's shadow.

A great advance in vision came with the development of eyes capable of collecting light and forming images on the array of photoreceptors. Although these eyes take many shapes throughout the animal kingdom,

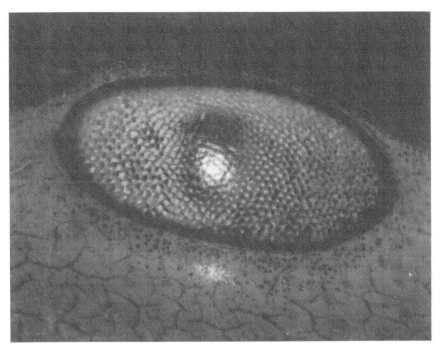

Figure 1.7. Lateral eye of *Limulus polyphemus*. The multiple facets of this compound eye are evident in the photograph. The central dark pseudopupil is caused by absorption of incident light within the ommatidia. (Reprinted, with permission, from W. W. Weiner and S. C. Chamberlain: The visual fields of American horseshoe crabs: two different eye shapes in *Limulus polyphemus*. *Visual Neuroscience* 11: 333–46, 1994.)

they can conveniently be divided into camera eyes and compound eyes. Camera eyes resemble photographic cameras in having a single chamber and an optical mechanism for forming an image of the outside world on a photosensitive surface, the retina. The camera eyes of invertebrates are often referred to as ocelli (singular, ocellus) and, sometimes, as simple eyes. The image-forming apparatus may be a tiny hole in the eyecup, resembling that of a pin-hole camera (Figure 1.6B), or some combination of a cornea and lens, such as occurs in vertebrates (Figure 1.6C). Compound eyes are found only in invertebrates and are composed of repeating modules called ommatidia, each with its own photoreceptors and imaging apparatus (Figures 1.6D and 1.7). In some compound eyes the adjacent ommatidia are optically isolated by pigment-containing cells; in others, an image is formed cooperatively by neighboring ommatidia.

Whereas vertebrates have only camera eyes, invertebrates can have both camera eyes and compound eyes. In addition to its two lateral compound eyes, *Limulus polyphemus*, the horseshoe crab, has four ocelli located in various places. Spiders and scorpions have 6–8 ocellar eyes, but no compound eyes. The scallop *Pecten* has about 60 simple eyes located along the edge of its mantle, which are of additional interest because they form images by reflection from a mirror-like structure behind the photoreceptors.

Eyes are composed of a variety of different tissues, brought together during development by a sequence of genetic signals that are still poorly understood. Important components of the vertebrate eye actually have their origin in the developing central nervous system and are incorporated into the peripheral organ of sight by a process of great complexity. In Chapter 2, we explore the basic components of the human eye and the processes that lead to its formation.

Further Reading

Goldsmith, T. H. (1990). Optimization, constraint, and history in the evolution of eyes. *Quarterly Review of Biology* 65:281–322.

Land, M. F. (1981). Optics and vision in invertebrates. In *Handbook of Sensory Physiology*, vol. 7, part 6B, ed. H. Autrum, pp. 471–592. Berlin: Springer-Verlag.

Land, M. F., and Fernald, R. D. (1992). The evolution of eyes. *Annual Review of Neuroscience* 15:1–29.

Nilsson, D.-E. (1990). From cornea to retinal image in invertebrate eyes. *Trends in Neurosciences* 13:55–64.

Wald, G. (1960). The distribution and evolution of visual systems. In *Comparative Biochemistry: A Comprehensive Treatise*, vol. 1, ed. M. Florkin and H. S. Mason, pp. 311–45. New York: Academic Press.

Walls, G. L. (1942). *The Vertebrate Eye and Its Adaptive Radiation*. New York: Hafner (reprinted 1963).

CHAPTER 2

STRUCTURE AND DEVELOPMENT OF THE HUMAN EYE

Major Anatomic Features of the Eye

Figure 2.1 illustrates schematically the major components of the human eye, which resembles that of most other primates. The sclera is a tough outer coat that is fibrous in humans but contains bone or cartilage in some other vertebrate species. The cornea is continuous with the sclera and provides the first element of the refracting media that bend the light to form an image on the retina. The lens lies behind the iris and in front of the vitreous humor, which fills the greater part of the globe. Aqueous humor fills the posterior chamber (the space between the lens and iris) and the anterior chamber (the space between the iris and the cornea). The posterior and anterior chambers are continuous through the pupil, the aperture formed by the iris.

The general features of the retina, the multilayered neural structure lining the back of the eyeball, can be visualized in the living eye with an ophthalmoscope or special camera (Figure 2.2). Axons leave the retina through the optic disc or optic papilla and enter the optic nerve to reach the brain. At the posterior pole of the eye, the retina thins to form the fovea, an area specialized for high-acuity vision. The visual axis is an imaginary line from the fovea through the center of the pupil (Figure 2.1). Behind the retina is the pigment epithelium, which is separated from the sclera by the vascular choroid. This vascular coat is continuous with similar

11

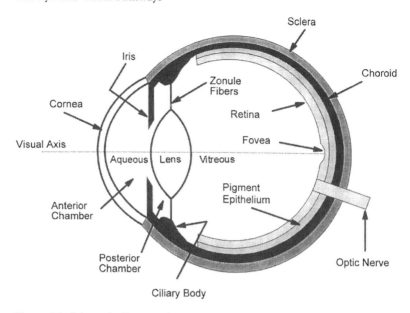

Figure 2.1. Schematic diagram of the major components of the human eye.

tissue of the ciliary body and the iris. The choroid and the fibrovascular components of the ciliary body and iris constitute the uvea. The retina and pigment epithelium originate from embryonic neural tissue that, as will be seen later, continues forward as a bilayered epithelium to cover the ciliary body and the posterior surface of the iris.

Animals whose survival depends on their ability to see in very dim light often have a mirror-like layer behind the retina that reflects light back through the photoreceptors (light that was not absorbed in its first pass). This layer, called a tapetum, may be a specialized region of the choroid or of the pigment epithelium, and its presence is responsible for the "eye-shine" that is seen when a car's headlights illuminate an animal at night. The tapetum of the domestic cat is formed by stacks of flat cells containing highly refractile rods and lying just behind the pigment epithelium. The presence of a tapetum obviously increases the overall sensitivity of the eye.

The ciliary body is a complex structure containing vascular tissue, muscle, and secretory epithelium. The ciliary muscle is involved in adjusting the shape of the lens, which is suspended in its capsule by the zonule fibers. The secretory epithelium produces the aqueous humor, which flows from the posterior chamber to the anterior chamber and then is emptied into the venous system.

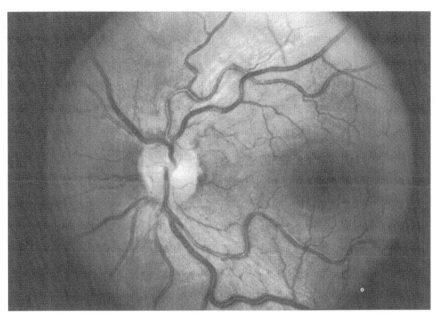

Figure 2.2. Fundus of the living human eye. The central retinal artery and vein are seen as they penetrate the optic disc. The fovea lies at the center of the macula lutea, the pigmented area to the right. (Courtesy of Dr. Caldwell Smith and Mark Hamel.)

The Vascular Supply of the Eye and the Blood–Ocular Barrier

Arterial blood reaches the orbit and the eye principally through the ophthalmic artery, which is the first intracranial branch of the internal carotid artery. Thus, when one examines the retinal arteries with an ophthalmoscope (Figure 2.2), one is looking directly at branches of an intracranial blood vessel. The uveal vasculature is fed by a family of ciliary arteries that are also branches of the ophthalmic artery. Some of these enter the eye around the margins of the optic disc, and others proceed to the anterior segment of the eye before penetrating the sclera.

The central retinal artery enters the eye through the optic disc and spreads its branches across the retina. After passing through the capillaries of the retina, the blood leaves through the central retinal vein and finds its way into the jugular vein and eventually back to the heart. Those vessels lying in the retina itself form the retinal circulation, which is to be distinguished from the choroidal circulation. The retinas of some animals contain no blood vessels and are said to be avascular. These retinas depend entirely on the choroid for their blood supply.

The human retina depends on both the choroid and the retinal vessels for its blood supply. These two vascular beds serve different parts of the retina and are regulated in different ways. The photoreceptors depend on the nearby choroid, which has a very high rate of blood flow that is determined principally by the arterial pressure. Because of the great metabolic needs of the photoreceptors, the eye seems to have adopted the strategy of "swamping" the choroid with blood to ensure that supply is never a problem. The choroidal blood flow is about 10 times that of a comparable volume of brain gray matter. The retinal vessels supply blood to the inner layers of the retina and are subject to a different kind of regulation ("inner" refers to the retinal layers closest to the center of the globe, and "outer" to those nearest the sclera). Here the flow rate is relatively independent of arterial pressure because the arterioles change their diameters in response to the metabolic needs of the local tissue. An increased need for oxygen or for removal of waste products results in dilation of the vessels and increased blood flow. This autoregulation of flow in the retinal vessels results from properties of the vascular smooth muscle itself, because the vessels are not innervated by the autonomic nervous system.

Blood flow to the eye not only supplies oxygen and nutrients but also removes aqueous humor and the waste products of metabolism and keeps the temperature of the eye within normal limits. Because the aqueous, vitreous, and lens are devoid of vessels, heat generated by metabolism or delivered directly into the eye by external sources (e.g., light, microwaves) can be removed only by blood flowing through the choroidal and retinal circulations. The former is clearly the more important because of the high rate at which blood flows through it. The rate of formation of aqueous and the maintenance of proper intraocular pressure also depend on precise regulation of blood flow to the eye.

The blood contains cellular elements and various substances that would interfere with retinal function if allowed to enter the neural tissue. A barrier to these is provided by tight junctions between cells of the retinal capillary walls that permit only certain constituents of plasma to cross into the retina itself. This system is in many ways analogous to the blood–brain barrier, which should come as no surprise, because the retina is a part of the brain stuck out on the end of the optic nerve. Large amounts of fluid leave the choroid, but the pigment epithelium stands between this flow and the retina and regulates the composition of materials reaching the retina. Similarly, large quantities of fluid must be provided through the ciliary processes in forming the aqueous humor, but the double-layered epithelium of the ciliary processes functions as a barrier to the passage of unwanted material. The anterior surface of the iris is devoid of epithelium, but its capillaries, like those of the retinal vessels, are provided with tight junctions that prevent leakage into the aqueous humor. Fine control of the composition of the fluid surrounding retinal elements and entering the aqueous humor depends on active transport of certain substances, such as glucose and key amino acids, that are needed to nourish the tissue.

The Tear Film

In many vertebrate eyes the first optical surface encountered by a light ray is the thin film of tears covering the cornea. This complex fluid has a critical optical function, in addition to other roles that it plays. The tear film of the human eye is composed of three distinct layers:

Superficial oily layer. This layer, only a few molecules thick at most, is formed from secretions of the Meibomian and sebaceous glands of the lids. It reduces evaporation from the underlying layers and forms a barrier near the lid margin to prevent tears from spilling onto the skin. In the absence of this layer, the evaporation rate of the tear film increases 10–20-fold. The oily layer forms the optical surface of the eye and ensures that this surface is as smooth as possible.

Lachrymal or tear fluid. This layer, 6.5–7.5 μm thick, is secreted by the main lachrymal gland and various accessory glands. Oxygen dissolved in this layer is available to the metabolic processes of the corneal epithelium. The lachrymal layer also provides a flushing action that removes foreign bodies from the cornea.

Mucoid layer. This very thin layer, secreted by goblet cells of the conjunctiva, serves as a wetting agent of the cornea. The corneal epithelium is hydrophobic; water does not wet it. The mucoid layer provides a hydrophilic layer over which the tear film can spread.

The tears are a solution of glucose, electrolytes, organic acids, enzymes, and other proteins. Some of the latter, including lysozyme and γ-globulins, provide an antibacterial action in the tear film. Blinking is important in maintaining the microstructure of the tear film. In the absence of blinking (such as occurs with facial nerve palsy and parkinsonism), the tear film tends to break up into patches, with consequent degradation of the optical qualities of the eye.

The Cornea

Figure 2.3 illustrates the main components of the cornea. It is covered in front by a multilayered epithelium that is continuous with the conjunctiva,

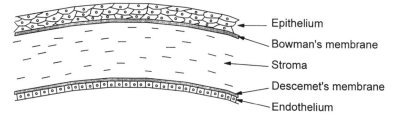

Figure 2.3. Diagrammatic cross section of the cornea.

which in turn is continuous with the skin. When damaged locally by a foreign body, the corneal epithelium surrounding the abrasion rapidly generates new cells that cover the injured area. The epithelium is separated from the stroma by Bowman's membrane, an acellular substance that cannot be separated from the stroma. The stroma, the thickest part of the cornea, is composed of collagen, mucopolysaccharides, and scattered cells called keratocytes. Descemet's membrane and the endothelium form the boundary between the stroma and the aqueous humor of the anterior chamber.

The corneal epithelium is supplied with free nerve endings from the trigeminal nerve. Because injury to the cornea is so painful, it once was thought that these nerve endings responded only to noxious stimuli. Subsequent research showed that they in fact respond to touch and pressure as well as to changes in temperature. The nerves responding to tactile stimulation participate in reflex circuits that cause rapid closing of the lids, the so-called corneal reflex. This reflex, which can be elicited by barely touching the cornea with a wisp of cotton, is clearly an important protective mechanism, providing a mechanical barrier to further injury. Activity in the same afferent fibers increases the production of tears, which, together with the movements of the lids, helps to remove debris from the corneal surface.

The cornea contains no blood vessels. The reasons for this are not clear, but there may be antivascular factors present in the tissue. The avascularity contributes to the optical clarity of the cornea, and because cellular elements involved in immune responses cannot reach the cornea through the blood, corneas can be transplanted from one person to another with considerable success.

The cornea is transparent when it is dehydrated. (The physical factors responsible for this will be discussed in Chapter 3.) Water is removed constantly from the corneal stroma by active transport mechanisms of the epithelium and endothelium, the latter transporting its volume of water every 5 minutes. These mechanisms require metabolic energy and involve active transport of ions. The energy required for this process is provided by nutrients in the aqueous humor. Oxygen from the air dissolves in the tear film and is also supplied from the aqueous humor. The cornea clouds if the eye is placed in an atmosphere of nitrogen. Evaporation of the tears also contributes to corneal dehydration by increasing the concentration of osmotically active components of the tear film. When the eyes are closed in sleep, this evaporation decreases, and slight swelling of the cornea occurs.

Injury to the endothelium or epithelium causes the cornea to imbibe water, to swell, and to become cloudy. This fact is exploited in diagnosing corneal abrasions due to foreign bodies or other trauma: A drop of a fluorescent substance in aqueous solution is placed on the eye and, where the epithelium is missing, is absorbed and concentrated in the stroma. After the excess dye is flushed from the cornea with water, examination with ultraviolet light reveals where the dye has remained at the site of the abrasion.

The Lens

The human lens has no blood supply, being dependent on nutrients from the aqueous humor. It is surrounded by a transparent capsule to which are attached the zonule fibers (Figure 2.4). These suspend the lens from the ciliary processes and posterior parts of the ciliary epithelium. The lens epithelium is present only at the anterior surface, for reasons that will be clear when we discuss the development of the eye. Throughout life, new lens fibers are added by dividing epithelial cells located on the margin or equator of the lens (Figure 2.4, right). No cells are lost from the lens during life.

Transparency of the lens depends on the presence of water-soluble proteins called crystallins in the lens fibers. The interiors of the lens fibers, like the cornea, must be maintained in a dehydrated state to support transparency. Maintenance of the crystallins also depends on active metabolic processes occurring principally in the nucleated cells of the epithelium and outer lamellae. Injury, infection, radiation, and metabolic diseases such as diabetes can cause lens opacifications called cataracts.

The Aqueous Humor and Intraocular Pressure

The pressure inside of the eyeball, normally about 15 mm Hg, maintains the shape of the eye and is crucial to its proper optical function. The pressure is determined by the rates of formation and egress of aqueous humor. The aqueous is formed in the frond-like ciliary processes of the

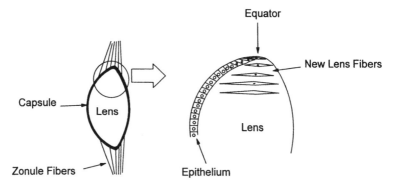

Figure 2.4. Structure of the lens. Left: The lens is suspended in its capsule by the zonule fibers. Right: Detail showing epithelium on anterior surface only and new lens fibers forming at the equatorial region. The thicknesses of the lens capsule and epithelium are highly exaggerated in this diagram.

ciliary body by a combination of plasma filtration, active transport, and secretion.

The aqueous humor circulates from the ciliary processes in the posterior chamber through the pupil and into the anterior chamber (Figure 2.5). It drains into the venous system through the canal of Schlemm, a channel in the corneal stroma that encircles the eye at the angle between the cornea and the iris, the so-called filtration angle. If the filtration angle is blocked by debris, bulging of the iris, or other pathological processes, egress of the aqueous humor is impaired, and the intraocular pressure rises. This condition is called glaucoma and is an important cause of blindness.

The Vitreous Humor

The vitreous humor fills the posterior part of the eyeball and serves to support the retina. Its major constituent is water, which provides a solvent for an assortment of ions and organic molecules. The water is constantly replaced by diffusion, largely from the aqueous humor. In humans, the liquid phase of the vitreous humor is weakly bound to a scaffolding of collagen fibrils, giving the vitreous humor the properties of a gel. In certain other animals the vitreous humor is a sol (i.e., the collagen fibrils are essentially suspended in the liquid phase). The vitreous humor is attached to the retina at its margin, around the optic disc and sometimes around the macula lutea, a pigmented area of the retina containing the fovea (Figure 2.2). Vitreal collapse sometimes occurs in the elderly or in those with

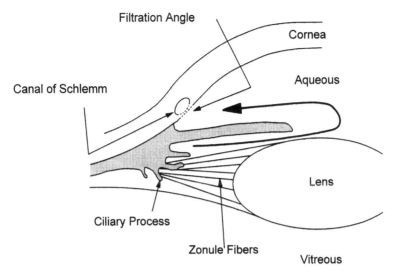

Figure 2.5. Circulation of the aqueous humor.

pathological conditions of the eye and can result in detachment and tearing of the retina.

Development of the Human Eye

The vertebrate nervous system develops from ectodermal tissue called the neural plate, located on the dorsal surface of the embryo. A depression, the neural groove, develops in this plate, and its lateral edges grow dorsally and approximate each other to fuse and form the neural tube. The lumen of the neural tube becomes the cerebral ventricles, cerebral aqueduct, and spinal canal. The brain and spinal cord develop from the walls of the neural tube. The eye begins to form as a bulge in the wall of that part of the neural tube destined to become the thalamus of the diencephalon. As this optic vesicle pushes toward the surface of the embryo, the overlying skin ectoderm begins to differentiate into the lens (Figure 2.6). The external surface of the optic vesicle is pushed back into the lumen to form a cup-like structure with inner and outer layers. The inner layer of the optic cup develops into the multilayered neural retina, and the sheet of cuboidal cells forming the outer layer becomes the pigment epithelium.

The space between the inner and outer layers of the optic cup is oblit-erated as the two layers contact one another, but it remains a virtual space throughout life. If bleeding or other injury occurs, the space can re-form

Optic Vesicle ⟶ Optic Cup

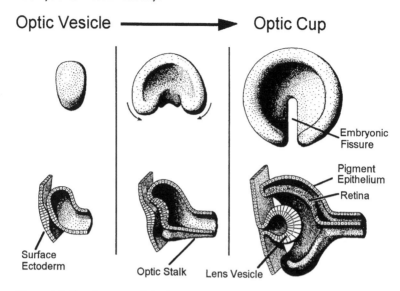

Figure 2.6. Development of the human eye. Three stages in the formation of the optic cup from the optic vesicle, seen face-on (top), and in cross section (bottom). Curved arrows in the top middle figure show how the margins of the invaginated vesicle approach each other inferiorly, leaving the embryonic fissure. The formation of the lens vesicle is also illustrated. (Adapted from G. L. Walls: *The Vertebrate Eye and Its Adaptive Radiation*. New York: Hafner. Copyright 1963, with permission of The Cranbrook Institute of Science.)

and push the retina away from the pigment epithelium, a situation called detached retina. Because the photoreceptors are nourished by blood vessels in the choroid, they cannot function when the retina detaches. The anterior lip of the optic cup later develops into the neural components of the iris, including two muscles, the sphincter pupillae and the dilator pupillae, that are unique in that they are muscles derived from neural ectoderm.

The tissue between the diencephalon and the eye is gradually modified to form the optic stalk, into which grow the axons of retinal ganglion cells on their way to the brain. Because of its embryonic connection to the brain, the optic nerve is covered with a tube of dura mater, and the interior of this tube remains in hydraulic continuity with the subarachnoid space, which contains the cerebrospinal fluid. Increased intracranial pressure can be communicated to the optic nerve and, if sustained, can damage the visual fibers within it, causing blindness.

As the optic cup forms, its rim does not immediately become perfectly circular, but rather exhibits a cleft near its inferior margin that extends all the way back to the site of the future optic disc (Figure 2.6). Into this embryonic fissure grow the primordial retinal vessels. As the margins of the fissure grow together and fuse to complete the lip of the optic cup, the retinal vessels are incorporated into the developing optic nerve and enter the eye at the optic disc (Figure 2.2).

During the early stages of the eye's development, these retinal vessels extend into the vitreous all the way to the lens, in addition to spreading across the retina itself. Toward the end of gestation, the vitreal branches of the retinal vessels are resorbed to leave the vitreous free of barriers to the passage of light. This same process leaves the vitreous and lens devoid of any direct vascular supply. When premature infants are placed temporarily in an atmosphere with a high oxygen concentration, because of the immaturity of their lungs, abnormal growth of the vascular and connective tissues of the retina may occur. This condition, retinopathy of prematurity, is a common cause of blindness in the newborn.

Development of the Lens, Cornea, and Sclera

As the optic vesicle approaches the skin or surface ectoderm, it sends a signal to that tissue that induces the formation of the lens. The skin first forms the lens vesicle, a hollow sphere that pinches off from the overlying ectoderm to lie within the rim of the optic cup (Figure 2.7). This process is enabled by earlier influences from foregut and heart mesoderm, so the process is very complex. The presence of the retina is essential for maintenance of the lens, which regresses if the retina is removed.

The ectodermal cells on the retinal side of the lens vesicle multiply and elongate into transparent lens fibers that eventually fill the lumen of the vesicle (Figure 2.7). As a result of this process, the original ectodermal layer remains only on the anterior surface of the lens and forms its epithelium. The orientation of the lens with respect to the optic axis is under exquisitely close control during development. If the lens is inverted experimentally, its internal structure becomes modified to restore the normal configuration. Fibers at the retinal pole elongate, old fibers recede, and new epithelium migrates over the corneal pole. This process is controlled by the neural retina, not by the cornea or sclera. The lens capsule is secreted by the lens epithelium, and the zonule fibers appear to be produced by the ciliary epithelium.

The stromal components of the cornea and sclera, as well as the corneal endothelium, develop from mesenchymal elements derived from the neural crest. The lens capsule appears to be the primary inducer of corneal differentiation. The corneal epithelium first differentiates where the lens capsule lies closest to the surface ectoderm. Then the stroma develops as layers

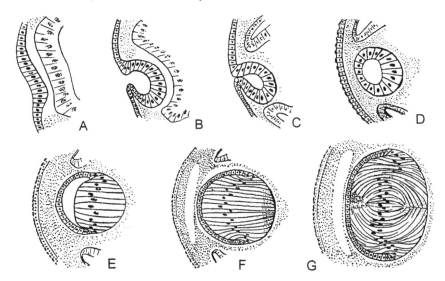

Figure 2.7. Development of the lens. (A–G) Sequential stages from lens vesicle to mature lens. (Reprinted from I. Mann: *The Development of the Human Eye*, 2nd ed. New York: Grune & Stratton. Copyright 1950, with permission of the British Medical Association.)

of evenly spaced collagen fibrils are laid down, each ply rotated about 45° with respect to its neighbor. The sequence of developmental steps, beginning with retinal induction of the lens and lens induction of the cornea, ensures that the optical elements of the eye are properly aligned with respect to the fovea.

Development of the Uvea and Associated Epithelia

The developmental relationship between eye and brain is strikingly illustrated in the disposition of their neural tissues and their fibrovascular coverings (Figure 2.8). In the eye, the fibrovascular choroid forms just outside the external layer of the optic cup (the future retinal pigment epithelium), just as the fibrous pia and its vessels envelop the external surface of the brain. In several places the brain tissue thins to a monolayer of epithelial cells that is invaginated by fibrovascular tissue to form the choroid plexus, source of the cerebrospinal fluid. With one slight difference, this same arrangement is found in the ciliary body of the eye. At

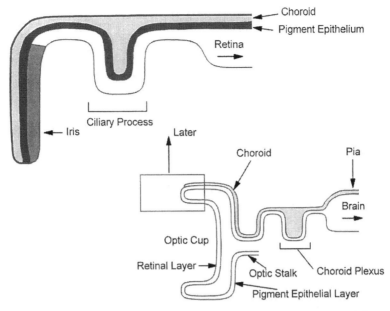

Figure 2.8. Schematic illustration of the analogous spatial relationships of fibro-vascular and neural tissues of brain and retina. Lower right: The rostral end of the neural tube forms the brain, the epithelium of the choroid plexus, and the optic cup. Apposed to these are fibrovascular tissues of the pia, the stroma of the choroid plexus, and the choroid, respectively. Upper left: Later in development, the inner (retinal) layer and outer (pigmented) layer of the optic cup fuse to form the two-layered epithelium covering the ciliary processes and the posterior surface of the iris. Apposed to this epithelium is a fibrovascular layer analogous to the choroid, the stroma of the choroid plexus, and the pia.

the margin of the optic cup the retinal layer thins and fuses with the pigmented outer layer of the cup. Vascularized connective tissue invaginates this bilayered epithelium to form the ciliary processes, which produce the aqueous humor. These same three elements continue toward the front of the eye, where they form the iris. In the iris, both layers of the bilayered epithelium become pigmented and lie on the retinal side of the fibrovascular stroma of the iris, which has no epithelium on its corneal side. Thus, the epithelium of the iris and ciliary body is the final product in the development of the anterior lip of the optic cup. The uvea (i.e., choroid and stromal elements of the ciliary body and iris) has its analogue in the pia of the brain and its associated blood vessels.

Development of the Retina

Retinal cellular proliferation begins at the ventricular face of the inner layer of the optic cup, leading first to a layer of primitive neuroepithelium (Figure 2.9). This layer thickens considerably as cell division continues, and a fibrous marginal layer appears toward the interior of the eye. Cells from the primitive cellular layer migrate into this region and form the inner neuroblastic layer. This layer subsequently splits, giving rise to the ganglion cell layer and the inner nuclear layer of the mature retina. Cells of the outer neuroblastic layer differentiate into the photoreceptors, whose cell bodies reside in the outer nuclear layer. A region of synaptic interaction, the inner plexiform layer, forms between the ganglion cell layer and inner nuclear layer. A similar zone, the outer plexiform layer, forms between the inner nuclear layer and the photoreceptor layer. Just as in the brain, cell differentiation occurs first in the layers farthest from the germinal layer. Thus, the first retinal cells to differentiate are the ganglion cells, which lie nearest the vitreous and send their axons into the optic nerve. The photoreceptors are the last to differentiate, and they remain next to the ventricle on the scleral (outer) side of the retina, adjacent to the pigment epithelium. This pattern of development explains why the vertebrate retina is inverted, in the sense that light must pass through several layers of the retina before reaching the photoreceptors.

There is also a developmental sequence that proceeds horizontally over time from the center of the retina to the periphery. Cellular differentiation begins near the future site of the fovea and progresses centrifugally across the retina toward its margin. As development continues, the total number of cells in the retina decreases, indicating that the final sculpting of connections and cell distributions involves programmed cell death. There is considerable variability in this process across vertebrate species. In some fish, for instance, photoreceptors are continuously added to the retina as the eye enlarges over the life of the animal.

Visual Experience and the Development of the Eye

It is apparent that the development of the eye is under exquisite genetic control to ensure that the several tissues involved in its formation differentiate in an orderly sequence and are properly positioned to effectively couple the optical and neural components. Not everything, though, is left to the control of the genetic program. The quality of the retinal image depends critically on the presence of a good match between the length of the eye and the optical power of its refracting elements (see Chapter 3), and the true test of this match cannot take place until the animal is born

Outer
Neuroblastic
Layer

Inner
Neuroblastic
Layer

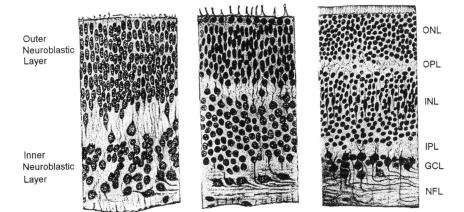

ONL

OPL

INL

IPL

GCL

NFL

Figure 2.9. Stages in the formation of the major layers of the human retina. The ventricular surface is at the top of the figure, and the vitreal surface at the bottom. The stratification of the mature retina is at the right. ONL, outer nuclear layer; OPL, outer plexiform layer; INL, inner nuclear layer; IPL, inner plexiform layer; GCL, ganglion cell layer; NFL, nerve-fiber layer. (Reprinted from B. M. Patten: *Human Embryology*, 2nd ed. New York: Blakiston. Copyright 1953, with permission of McGraw-Hill, Inc.)

and its eyes are open. Thus, it would be advantageous to fine-tune the relationship between optical power and eye size to obtain the sharpest possible image after the eye is exposed to real stimuli. Studies in several species indeed suggest that the quality of the retinal image can influence the size of the eye in young animals.

T. N. Wiesel and E. Raviola first showed that occlusion of one eye by lid suture in infant macaque monkeys caused that eye to grow in length. This phenomenon, called deprivation myopia, has subsequently been demonstrated in a number of other species using various methods to blur the retinal image. The changes in the retina are regional, in that blurring of part of the retinal image in the chick leads to excessive growth only in that part of the eye deprived of pattern stimulation. Deprivation-induced changes in axial length will occur in some species after sectioning of the optic nerve, suggesting that there are local mechanisms by which the retina can detect blurring and modify the length of the eye. There is as yet no satisfactory answer to the question of how the retina senses the sharpness of the image imposed upon it, but a burgeoning field of research is assessing the roles of accommodation, intraocular pressure, choroidal blood flow, corneal flattening, and a number of humoral factors in the response to image blurring.

Further Reading

Bock, G., and Widdows, K. (eds.) (1990). *Myopia and the Control of Eye Growth.* Ciba Foundation Symposium 155. New York: Wiley.

Browder, L. W. (1984). *Developmental Biology*, 2nd ed. Philadelphia: Saunders.

Carp, G., and Berrill, N. J. (1981). *Development*, 2nd ed. New York: McGraw-Hill.

Coulombre, A. J. (1965). The eye. In *Organogenesis*, ed. R. L. DeHaan and H. Ursprung, pp. 219–51. New York: Holt, Rinehart & Winston.

Moses, R. A., and Hart, W. M., Jr. (1987). *Adler's Physiology of the Eye*, 8th ed. St. Louis: Mosby.

Wiesel, T. N., and Raviola, E. (1977). Myopia and eye enlargement after neonatal lid suture in monkeys. *Nature* 266:66–88.

CHAPTER 3

IMAGE FORMATION

This chapter introduces certain physical principles that are important to an understanding of how images are formed by optical systems. We then treat the structures and mechanisms in the human eye that produce the retinal image and determine its quality.

It is useful to begin by briefly discussing light as an oscillating electromagnetic field, because many properties of optical systems such as that of the eye depend on the nature of these fields. An electromagnetic field arises from the motion of a charge and propagates away in all directions perpendicular to the charge's axis of movement. Figure 3.1A illustrates this schematically for a charge oscillating sinusoidally in the plane of the page. The sinusoidal wave depicted represents only the electric field produced by the moving charge; at right angles to the electric field, normal to the plane of the page, is an oscillating magnetic field. Seen from above (Figure 3.1B), the electromagnetic field, represented here by the positive peaks of its electric component, propagates away from the charge as a succession of curved wave fronts that can be treated as planar at some distance from the source (right side of Figure 3.1B). Depending on the situation, it is convenient to think of light either as an advancing wave front or as a ray, the latter usually being represented by an arrow normal to the advancing wave front.

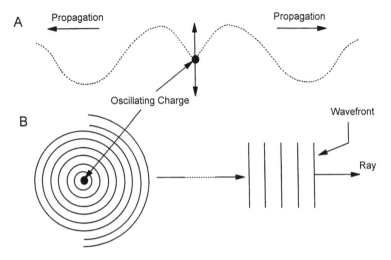

Figure 3.1. Generation and propagation of an electromagnetic field. (A) A moving charge generates an electromagnetic field that propagates away in all directions at right angles to the direction of motion of the charge. If the charge moves sinusoidally, the field also varies sinusoidally in time and space. One cycle of the sinusoid defines its period, P; the frequency of the sinusoid is $1/P$. In angular units, a period contains 360°, and any position along the wave front can be specified by its phase, i.e., its displacement in degrees from some reference point on the wave. (B) Here the charge is depicted as moving normal to the plane of the page, and the positive peaks of its generated field are illustrated as concentric circles. At a distance from the moving charge, the circles expand sufficiently that, locally, the waveform can be approximated by a plane.

Scatter, Interference, and Transparency

When a propagating wave front of light encounters matter, charges in the matter experience the alternating electromagnetic field, and some are set in motion. These moving charges then give rise to their own oscillating electromagnetic fields, which propagate away as in Figure 3.1. This phenomenon is called scatter. When the moving charges are not densely packed and are distributed in a more or less random fashion, the combined fields of all the charges exit the medium in various directions, and the medium looks cloudy.

The multitude of new fields generated by the moving charges interact with each other within the medium. This interaction or interference is additive or constructive when the fields at a given point in space are of the same sign, and subtractive or destructive when some of the fields are positive and others are negative (Figure 3.2A). Because the net field at any one point in the medium is the sum of all the fields interacting at that

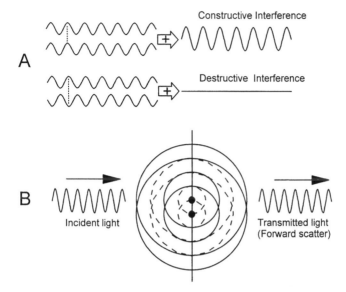

Figure 3.2. Schematic illustration of interference and forward scattering. (A) Sinusoidal waves traveling to the right sum when their positive peaks are aligned at a point in space (top pair) and cancel when the positive peaks of one align with the negative peaks of the other (bottom pair). The former is called constructive interference, and the latter destructive interference. The sign and degree of such interference vary as the degree of alignment, or relative phase, of the waves varies. (B) These two charges spaced one-half wavelength apart (180° spatial phase) oscillate normal to the page and in temporal phase. Positive peaks are shown as solid circles, and negative peaks as dashed circles. The generated fields interfere constructively in the direction of the incident light, where peaks of the same sign align, and destructively at right angles to this, along a line through the charges where the peaks of different sign align. In a transparent substance, light scattered back toward the incident light undergoes destructive interference. Any that persists is said to be reflected.

point, wherever the sum of negative voltages equals the sum of positive voltages the field is cancelled. A medium becomes transparent when all the fields due to scatter cancel except those propagating in one direction, called the direction of forward scatter. This is usually the direction of the incident light.

For this direction-specific cancellation to occur, neighboring charges must have a certain geometric relationship to each other, as illustrated schematically in Figure 3.2B. Here, two charges separated by half a wavelength of light and seen from above are moving in and out of the page together (i.e., in temporal phase). Observe that along a line drawn through the two charges the positive peaks of the field produced by one charge (solid circles) occur at the negative peaks produced by the other (dashed circles). If more charges are added between the two original ones and out along that same line in both directions, a situation exists in which for every charge there is another whose field exactly cancels that of the first. However, in a direction at right angles to the line through the two charges in Figure 3.2B, the peaks and troughs reinforce each other. The net field from a line of such charges is strongest in this direction and is zero along the line through the charges. In a transparent substance, the affected charges are separated from each other in three dimensions by distances smaller than the wavelength of the incident light, so that mutual interference between neighboring oscillators cancels all scattered fields except those moving in the direction of the incident light, the direction of forward scatter.

Thus, a substance is transparent if it has the property that only forward scatter survives the interference among the secondary waves produced by the moving charges within it. Transparency of the cornea and lens is based on this property. Dehydration of the cornea creates the geometric relationships required for transparency by forcing the scattering elements (i.e., the collagen fibrils) into close proximity with each other. When the cornea imbibes water, the fibrils are forced apart, and scattered light begins to emerge from the cornea in all directions. Similarly, transparency of the lens depends on maintaining its constituent crystallin proteins at a concentration sufficiently high that light scattered laterally from them undergoes destructive interference. When a cataract forms because of disease or physical injury, scattered light emerges from the lens in all directions.

The kind of scatter just described is called elastic scatter, because no energy is extracted from the incident field. Light can also be absorbed by a medium, setting its constituent atoms and molecules into motion and raising the temperature of the medium. The energy converted to heat is lost by the incident light.

Refraction and the Refractive Index

It is evident from the preceding discussion that light does not simply pass through a transparent medium, but actually interacts with it in a complex fashion. In fact, the incident light experiences interference with the secondary waves arising from the very charges it has set in motion, and these secondary waves produce yet further motions in other charges, and so on. One consequence of this complex pattern of destructive and constructive interference is that the wave front appears to propagate more slowly in matter than it does in a vacuum. The degree of slowing varies with the nature of the matter and with the wavelength of the light, shorter wavelengths being affected more than longer.

Light propagates through a vacuum at 3×10^8 m/s, a universal constant designated c, and when it enters another medium its progress slows to some speed v. The ratio c/v is the index of refraction, n, of the medium and is always greater than or equal to 1. In air, v differs so little from c that the refractive index of air is usually taken to be 1.0. The refractive index of water is about 1.3, and that of silicate crown glass about 1.5. Strictly speaking, though, one should specify the wavelength for which a particular refractive index applies, as the degree of slowing is greater for short than for long wavelengths. It is evident from the definition of n that light propagates at different speeds though media having different indices of refraction. Often associated with this change in speed is a change in direction, which provides the basis for image formation in most eyes.

Why Does Light Bend When It Passes from One Medium to Another with a Different Index of Refraction?

One way to understand this is to begin with Huygens's principle, which states that every point on a wave front advancing through a particular medium at speed v is the origin of a secondary wavelet that also propagates at speed v (Figure 3.3). After some interval of time t, the wave front is located at a surface tangent to the expanding wavelets and has advanced a distance vt.

Consider now, in Figure 3.4A, the segment AB of a wave front in air ($n = 1$) as it approaches a plane glass surface ($n' = 1.5$) in the direction of the arrows. We assume that the wave front is sufficiently far from the light source that it can be considered planar. At the instant when point A touches the glass, let a secondary wavelet emerge and travel through the glass at the lower speed v'. At the same instant a secondary wavelet at point B emerges, advances through air at speed v, and reaches the glass at point D after t seconds. During this interval the wavelet from point A, moving more slowly, has reached point C in the glass. Note that in time t the wavelet from B travels farther than that from A. Because a similar phenomenon happens continuously along the surface, by the end of interval t the wave front is at CD, and its direction of propagation has changed.

Wave segment AB makes angle θ_i, and CD makes angle θ_r, with the glass surface in Figure 3.4A. Note that $\angle ABD$ and $\angle ACD$ are right angles.

$$\sin \theta_i = vt/AD \quad \text{and} \quad \sin \theta_r = v't/AD, \quad \text{so} \quad \sin \theta_i/\sin \theta_r = v/v'.$$

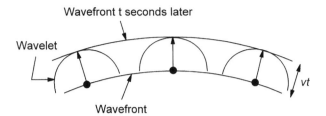

Figure 3.3. Huygens's principle. Each point on the expanding wave front is assumed to give rise to a wavelet that sums with those from adjacent points to move the wave front forward. If the light propagates at velocity v, the front advances a distance of vt in time t.

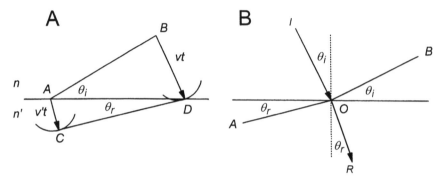

Figure 3.4. Geometry of Snell's law. Refraction at a planar surface.

Because $n = c/v$ and $n' = c/v'$,

$$\sin \theta_i / \sin \theta_r = n'/n \quad \text{or} \quad n \sin \theta_i = n' \sin \theta_r. \tag{1}$$

It is easier to deal with the phenomenon of refraction in terms of light rays, which can be thought of as normal to the plane of the wave front (arrows in Figure 3.4B). Consider the situation when wave front AB of Figure 3.4A has passed halfway into the glass (Figure 3.4B). The wave front is bent at point O because the part inside the glass is traveling more slowly than the part still in air. The incident ray IO and the refracted ray OR are deviated from a normal to the glass surface (dotted line) by the same angles, θ_i and θ_r, respectively, that describe the deviations of the two halves of the wave front from the glass surface. Angle θ_i of Figure 3.4B is called the angle of incidence, and angle θ_r the angle of refraction. The relationship involving θ_i, θ_r, n, and n' given in equation (1) is called Snell's law.

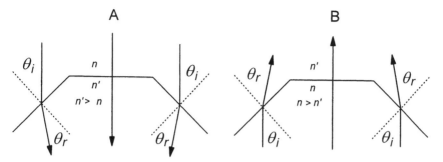

Figure 3.5. Refraction at a nonplanar surface.

Note that refraction occurs when the speed of light changes as it passes from one medium into another. Thus, the amount of bending is not a function of the absolute value of the refractive index of either medium, but rather of the change in refractive index as the light crosses an interface between two media. This is illustrated by the fact that some clear plastics have refractive indices so close to that of water that when they are immersed they are no longer visible. As shown later, the contribution of the human lens to the refractive power of the eye is relatively small, because its refractive index is not much different from that of the fluid surrounding it.

How Does the Curvature of a Surface Affect the Bending of Light Rays?

According to Snell's law, $\sin \theta_r = (n/n')\sin \theta_i$, so if $n' > n$, then θ_r, the angle of refraction, will be smaller than θ_i, the angle of incidence. This fact is useful in understanding the next point. Also, note that by convention the refractive index of the first medium through which the light passes is designated n, the second n', the third n'', and so forth.

Consider a glass surface presenting three plane facets to a bundle of parallel rays (a planar wave front) advancing through air (Figure 3.5A). The dashed lines are normal to the facets. The middle ray is normal to the surface of the middle facet, so it is not bent ($\sin \theta_i = 0$, so $\sin \theta_r$ must also equal zero). The left and right rays are bent toward the middle ray, because in both cases $n' > n$, so $\theta_r < \theta_i$. The same would occur if the surface were smoothly curved, in which case normals to the surface would vary continuously in orientation instead of abruptly as in Figure 3.5. Increasing the curvature of the surface would increase the convergence effect.

Figure 3.5A shows that rays converge when they move across a convex surface into a medium of higher refractive index. Rays approaching the same surface from inside the medium of higher refractive index also con-

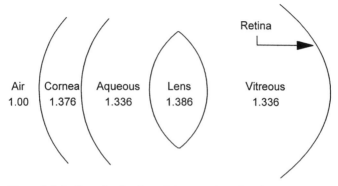

Figure 3.6. Indices of refraction of the optical media of the human eye.

verge, because in this case $n > n'$ and $\theta_r > \theta_i$ (Figure 3.5B). Thus, rays converge when they move in either direction across a surface that is convex toward the medium of lower refractive index, and by analogous arguments they diverge when they cross a surface that is concave toward the medium of lower refractive index. Therefore, whether rays converge or diverge when they pass from one medium into another depends on two factors: (1) the change in refractive index and (2) the curvature of the interface between the two media.

Figure 3.6 compares the refractive indices of the ocular media through which rays of light must pass to reach the human retina. Because the degree of bending is a function of the difference between the refractive indices of two media, it is clear that the greatest contribution to the human eye's optical power comes from the air–cornea interface. Immersion of the cornea in water greatly reduces its contribution to the eye's power, which is why a person under water cannot see objects clearly unless a face mask is used to restore the air–cornea interface. Note that at the cornea–aqueous interface, light rays encounter a concave surface facing a medium of lower refractive index, and consequently they diverge.

Because the air–cornea interface is so important optically, uniformity in both its surface and curvature is absolutely crucial to good image formation. Scarring of the cornea or asymmetries of curvature substantially reduce image quality. These anomalies may completely incapacitate the eye, whereas the small loss of power due to lens extraction can be overcome by spectacles, contact lenses, or, now, intraocular lens implants.

The Thin Lens

Many of the principles governing image formation in the eye are illustrated by the properties of a lens of negligible thickness. Rays striking the lens

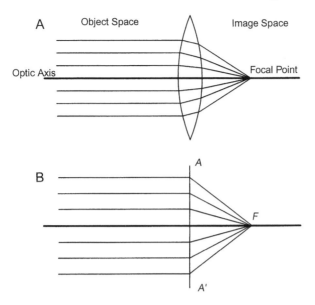

Figure 3.7. Thin biconvex lens in air. AA', the lens plane; F, focal point.

of Figure 3.7A are rendered convergent by both surfaces because of the principles just stated. If the lens is very thin, it is possible to ignore its thickness and assume that all rays are bent at a plane perpendicular to the optic axis of the lens and located at its center (the lens plane, AA' in Figure 3.7B). The parallel rays striking the lens converge toward a point F on the axis called the focal point of the lens. Another definition of the focal point is that point on the axis from which emerging rays are rendered parallel by the lens. Because the light can come from either direction, there are focal points on either side of the lens. The distance from the plane AA' to the focal point is the focal length of the lens. With the thin lens in air, the focal lengths on the two sides are equal. (Caveat: These notions and those discussed later assume also that the rays strike the lens close to the lens axis, i.e., that they are paraxial rays. Certain optical aberrations discussed later arise because not all rays obey these rules exactly.)

An object located, say, to the left of the lens (in object space) is imaged somewhere to the right of the lens (in image space). For this to happen, though, the object must lie farther from the lens than the focal length. It is easy to understand why this is true, because rays diverging from a point nearer to the lens than the primary focal point are not bent sufficiently to render them parallel, much less convergent.

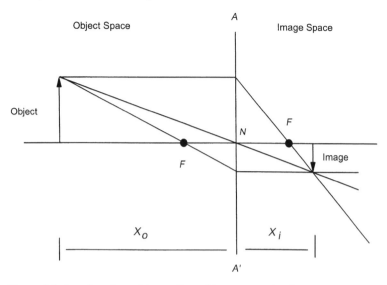

Figure 3.8. Locating the real image formed by a converging lens.

The position of the image formed by a thin lens can be found if the focal length is known, as shown in the construction of Figure 3.8. The tail of the arrow in object space is on the optic axis at the left and is imaged somewhere on the same axis to the right of the lens in image space. A line from the head of the arrow parallel to the axis passes through the focal point in image space. A line from the head of the arrow through the center of the lens (a central ray) is not deviated. The intersection of these last two lines gives the position of the image of the arrowhead. Alternatively, a ray from the arrowhead through the focal point to the left of the lens in object space is rendered parallel to the axis and intersects one of the other lines at the location of the image. Using any two of the three lines does the trick. This image is inverted and real, the latter referring to the fact that the image appears on a piece of paper placed in the image plane. The location of the image depends on the focal length of the lens and the distance of the object from the lens. The tips of the arrowheads in object and image are said to be conjugate points of the optical system, and the planes in which object and image lie are conjugate planes. Point N at the center of this thin lens is the nodal point, defined as a point in the optical system through which rays pass without changing direction. Knowing where this point is located in the eye is important, as we shall see.

The ratio of image size to object size is the magnification of the object.

How much an object is magnified depends on its distance from the lens and the focal length of the lens. Observe that the size of the image can be obtained from the geometrical relations of Figure 3.8 if the distances x_o and x_i and the size of the object are known. By similar triangles, object/image = x_o/x_i. This relationship becomes important when we wish to know the sizes of retinal images.

Lenses of shorter focal lengths have greater refractive power than lenses of longer focal lengths. In order that lens power be expressed as a number that increases with refractive capacity, it is defined as the reciprocal of the focal length in meters: $P = 1/f$. The unit of refracting power is the diopter (D). A lens with a focal length of 0.5 m has a power of 2 diopters, or 2 D. The power of the human eye is about 60 D, of which about 45 D is contributed by the cornea. The lens contributes another 15 D or so.

Estimating Image Size in the Eye

A key feature of the situation shown in Figure 3.8 is that a ray of light passing through the center of the thin lens does not change direction. The human eye, however, contains more than one refracting element and thus is a compound optical system. Such systems do not have a single nodal point, but it is possible to identify two theoretical points on the optic axis that have the property that a ray drawn from an object to the first point can be considered to exit the second point in the same direction (Figure 3.9A). In the human eye, the posterior nodal point of the eye (N_p in Figure 3.9A) is located near the back of the lens and lies about 15–17 mm in front of the retina. This separation is called the posterior nodal distance (PND) and varies slightly from person to person. The anterior nodal point (N_a in Figure 3.9A) is about 0.25 mm anterior to the posterior nodal point.

Figure 3.9B shows a simplification that makes it easy to estimate the size of a retinal image under conditions of normal viewing. Because the distance between the two nodal points is usually small relative to the distance from the eye to the object, it can be ignored and the eye can be considered to have only one nodal point (N in Figure 3.9B), located at the position of the posterior nodal point (i.e., about 17 mm in front of the human retina). Similarly, because the distance d from the posterior nodal point to the front of the cornea is small relative to the distance from N to the object, it, too, can be ignored, and the distance $x + d$ can be taken as equal to x. A ray from the head of the arrow of height y in Figure 3.9B is drawn to the nodal point, making an angle θ with the optic axis. This ray emerges from the nodal point in the same direction (at the same angle with respect to the axis) and intersects the retina at the location of the

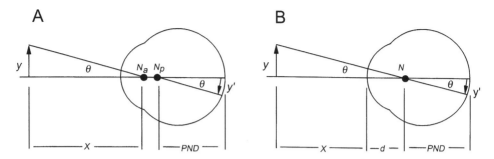

Figure 3.9. Calculating image size in the eye. (A) Compound optical systems, such as the eye, have two nodal points. (B) A simplified scheme with one nodal point (N) to facilitate calculation of retinal-image size. N_a, anterior nodal point; N_p, posterior nodal point; N, schematic nodal point of simplified system; PND, posterior nodal distance; d, distance from N to anterior corneal surface; y, height of object; y', height of retinal image.

arrowhead's image. The height of the arrow y can be stated in terms of the angle θ, which is

$$\theta = \tan^{-1} (y/x) \ [y/x \text{ is essentially the same as } y/(x + d)].$$

The height of the retinal image $y' = (\text{PND}) \cdot \tan \theta = (\text{PND}) \cdot (y/x)$.

The angle θ is said to be the visual subtense of the object in visual angle or visual arc. It is useful to express performance measures such as visual acuity in terms of visual angle rather than absolute spatial units, so that the measure is independent of object distance.

Example. How high is the retinal image of a 6-foot-tall man standing 20 feet from an observer whose PND is 17 mm? We have $y = 6$ feet, $x = 20$ feet, PND = 17 mm. Note that because we use the ratio y/x, their units disappear in the calculation.

$$y' = (\text{PND}) \cdot (y/x) = (17 \text{ mm})(6/20) = 5.1 \text{ mm}.$$

Diverging Lenses and Virtual Images

The thin lens of Figure 3.10 is said to be biconcave because it presents concave surfaces to the air on both sides. Because of relationships described earlier, a bundle of parallel rays striking this lens from either side will diverge and not be gathered into a real image. However, when these di-

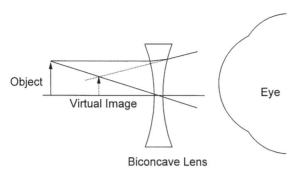

Figure 3.10. Diverging lenses and virtual images.

verging rays enter the eye, the high power of the eye's optics can sometimes cause them to converge to form a real image on the retina. The
brain interprets these rays as diverging from a small object located on the
other side of the lens and closer to the eye than the real object. Because
this image will not form on a piece of paper held anywhere in object or
image space, it is called the virtual image of the real object. The location
of this virtual image can be found by procedures analogous to those described earlier for the biconvex lens, but these will not be detailed here.
Because the virtual image formed by a diverging lens is located in object
space, the lens is said to have a negative focal length and negative refractive
power. For instance, a lens of −2 D refractive power will make parallel
rays seem to arise from a point 0.5 m from the lens in object space.
Diverging lenses are commonly called "minus" lenses, and converging
lenses "plus" lenses.

Spectacle Lenses

If you examine your own or your neighbor's eyeglasses you will note that
they are neither biconvex nor biconcave, but rather combine a convex
anterior surface with a concave posterior surface. These are called concavo-
convex lenses or meniscus lenses. The power of such a lens can be adjusted
for positive or negative values by varying the curvatures of the anterior
and posterior surfaces. In principle, one can make lenses with only one
curved surface. Such plano-convex and plano-concave lenses are not ordinarily used for spectacles, but are found in microscopes and other types of
optical instruments.

Lens Aberrations

An ideal lens would reproduce each point on an object as a point in the
image, but this does not happen because of certain inherent physical prop-

erties of light and lenses. Light from a point in the object generally forms a blur circle in the image. The deviations of a lens from ideal performance are called aberrations, and there are two major classes: chromatic and monochromatic.

Chromatic aberration. Consider a white object point located a great distance from the lens, but on its axis. Light emerging from this point contains all visible wavelengths. Now, because the refractive index of a medium depends on wavelength, the different components of the white light emerging from this point are refracted to different degrees, and the various chromatic components are strewn along the axis in image space (Figure 3.11A). Red light is bent less than blue light, so the red component of the image lies farthest from the lens. This is axial chromatic aberration. By the same token, regions of an object off the axis have the red points displaced laterally with respect to the blue points in the image. This is lateral chromatic aberration. In fact, the distant white point giving rise to the parallel rays is not imaged on a plane, but in a volume of image space. This obviously degrades the image. There are various ways of correcting for chromatic aberration in lenses, such as by combining two kinds of glass of different refractive indices and appropriate curvatures, so that their chromatic aberrations cancel each other.

Monochromatic aberrations. Certain defects in images formed by lenses arise from systematic variations in the amounts of bending that occur across a curved refracting surface, variations resulting from an interplay between the changing angle of incidence and the refractive power of the surface. These appear even when monochromatic light is used to produce the image. As an example, when parallel rays from a distant point reach a spherical refracting surface, rays striking the periphery of the lens are bent more than those passing through its center (Figure 3.11B). This spherical aberration prevents points on the object from being imaged as perfect points in the image. Other monochromatic aberrations also contribute geometric imperfections to the image, but they need not concern us here. What is important is that because these phenomena are most pronounced when light strikes a large area of a curved refracting surface, they can be reduced by restricting the bundle of rays to those traveling close to the axis of the lens.

Refractive Errors of the Eye

The human eye can change its refractive power by varying the curvature of the lens. When the muscles that do this are paralyzed, most human

A

Chromatic Aberration

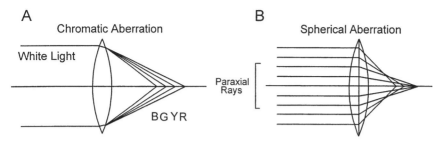

White Light

BG Y R

B

Spherical Aberration

Paraxial
Rays

Figure 3.11. Chromatic aberration and spherical aberration. (A) The image of a white point is strewn along the lens axis, because short wavelengths are bent more than long wavelengths. B, blue; G, green; Y, yellow; R, red. (B) Rays far from the lens axis are bent more than paraxial rays, resulting in spherical aberration.

eyes image parallel rays on the retina, as though the retina contained the focal point of the optical system under these conditions. This situation is called emmetropia, which is from the Greek *en* (in) and *metron* (measure). Refractive errors arise from mismatches between the refractive power of the eye and its length, or because of abnormal corneal curvature (Figure 3.12). As just noted, an emmetropic eye that cannot accommodate because of paralysis of the ciliary muscle focuses parallel incident rays on the retina. In myopia, the image forms in front of the retina, usually because the eyeball is abnormally long (axial myopia), but sometimes because the dioptrics are too powerful. Myopia is corrected by introducing diverging or minus lenses in the optic path. Myopia is commonly referred to as near-sightedness, because image clarity is improved by bringing an object closer to the eye, and thus moving the image toward the retina. In hypermetropia, the image forms behind the retina because the eyeball is too short. Hypermetropia, sometimes called hyperopia or farsightedness, is corrected with converging or plus lenses.

Another common refractive error, astigmatism, is best understood by considering those planes through a lens that contain the lens axis (Figure 3.13). These are called meridional planes, because their intersections with a sphere would mark great circles corresponding to meridians of longitude. If the lens is more steeply curved along one meridian than along the others, the rays of light aligned with that meridian are focused closer to the lens than other rays. The lens of Figure 3.13 has a steeper curvature along its horizontal meridian than along its vertical meridian. As the lens intercepts a bundle of parallel rays from some distant point, those rays lying in the horizontal plane (stippled) are bent more than those in the vertical plane and come to a focus closer to the lens. The image of this point, then, lies

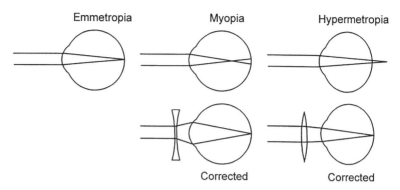

Figure 3.12. Refractive errors of the eye.

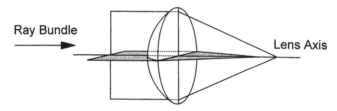

Figure 3.13. Astigmatism due to aspherical curvature. This plano-convex lens is curved more strongly along its horizontal meridian than along its vertical meridian. Rays encountering the horizontal meridian are focused in front of those refracted along the vertical meridian.

not in a plane, but along the lens axis. Were the object a two-dimensional one, its image would occupy a volume rather than a plane.

The most common cause of astigmatism in the human eye is non-sphericity of the cornea. Spectacles designed to correct for astigmatism combine a cylindrical lens that has refractive power only along one dimension (to balance out the asymmetry of the cornea) with a spherical lens to correct other errors. Such a combination is called a toric lens.

Effect of the Pupil

It has already been emphasized that the effects of many lens aberrations can be reduced by restricting the bundle of rays to those near the lens axis. This applies to the eye as well, and a major function of the iris

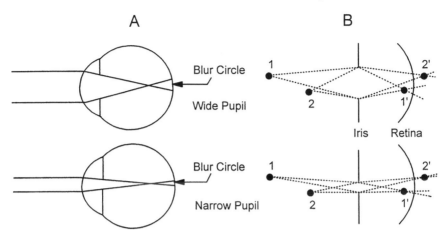

Figure 3.14. Effects of pupil diameter on blur-circle size and depth of field.

muscles is to narrow the pupil so as to exclude peripheral rays. The combined effects of aberrations and refractive errors cause rays from a point in an object to converge to a blur circle on the retina. Figure 3.14A shows how exclusion of the peripheral rays narrows the size of the blur circle due to myopia. When the blur circles become small enough, the retina cannot distinguish them from true points.

Pupil diameter, through its effect on blur-circle size, also influences the depth of field of the eye, that is, the range of distances over which objects produce clear images on the retina for a given state of accommodation. Observe that the point objects 1 and 2 in Figure 3.14B produce large blur circles on the retina because of the dilated pupil. When the pupil constricts, the blur circles decrease in size, and the images of points 1 and 2 become sharper.

One might think that a very narrow pupil would be the best, but reducing pupil diameter below about 2 mm causes the image to degrade because of diffraction. This phenomenon, which is not the same as refraction, originates in the wave nature of light and the ability of light wavelets to cancel or interfere with each other. Diffraction effects are introduced by edges (like the edge of the iris) in the light path and cause a certain amount of blur in the image. It suffices here to point out that such effects are always present in the retinal image, but when the pupil is large they are relatively insignificant. As the pupil constricts, diffraction makes a larger contribution to the distribution of light in the image, and at diameters less than 2 mm it becomes the major factor reducing image sharpness.

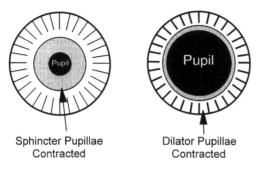

Figure 3.15. Geometry of the sphincter and dilator muscles of the human iris. Contraction of the sphincter pupillae reduces the diameter of the pupil (left), and contraction of the dilator pupillae increases it (right).

Pupil diameter is decreased by contraction of the sphincter pupillae muscle, which rings the inner edge of the iris (Figure 3.15, left). The sphincter pupillae is a smooth muscle innervated by the parasympathetic system. Preganglionic cells in the Edinger-Westphal nucleus send their axons to the ciliary ganglion, where postganglionic cholinergic cells in turn project through ciliary nerves to the iris. Constriction of the pupil is called miosis, and drugs that cause constriction are called miotics. These act usually by imitating acetylcholine or by blocking its inactivation.

Dilation of the pupil results from contraction of the dilator pupillae, a smooth muscle innervated by the sympathetic nervous system (Figure 3.15, right). Sympathetic preganglionic cells of the spinal cord send their axons into the sympathetic trunk, where they synapse in the superior cervical ganglion. From there, postganglionic adrenergic fibers proceed in the carotid plexus to join the ciliary nerves that supply the iris. Dilation of the pupil is called mydriasis, and drugs causing dilation are called mydriatics. These act by imitating the action of norepinephrine or by blocking the action of acetylcholine and relaxing the sphincter pupillae.

Accommodation

Accommodative mechanisms adjust the optical system of the eye to form crisp retinal images of objects located different distances away. Very small eyes require little accommodative capacity because they focus virtually all images over a range of retinal depths that are short relative to the lengths of the photoreceptors. In larger terrestrial animals, accommodation for near objects requires that the lens curvature increase or that the lens move away from the retina.

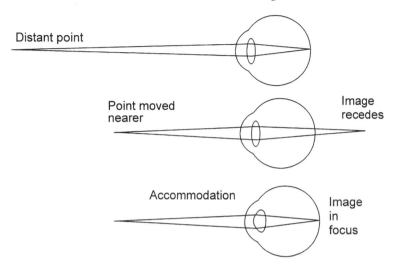

Figure 3.16. Role of the lens in accommodation. Increased curvature of the lens results in greater optical power and a decrease in the effective focal length of the eye. This serves to position the image of a near object in the plane of the retina.

As an object moves nearer to the eye, its image tends to recede behind the retina (Figure 3.16). In the primate eye, accommodation for near objects requires that the optical power of the lens increase to reduce the effective focal length of the eye and bring the image forward to the plane of the retina. In humans and other primates, the lens is enclosed in its capsule, which is suspended behind the iris by zonule fibers attached to the ciliary body (Figures 2.1 and 3.17). The zonule fibers maintain a constant tension on the rim of the capsule, and this tends to flatten the pliable lens. The zonule fibers are attached to the ciliary body, which forms a ring around the lens, and within the ciliary body there is a set of smooth muscle fibers that encircle the lens like a sphincter (Figure 3.17). When these ciliary-muscle fibers contract, the diameter of the ring of attachment of the zonule fibers decreases, the tension on the fibers is relieved, and the lens surfaces become more curved. Other parts of the ciliary muscle pull the attachments of the zonule fibers forward, an action that also reduces the tension on the fibers and the capsule.

In a young person, contraction of the ciliary muscle and rounding of the lens can increase the optical power of the eye by about 14 D. As an individual ages, new fibers are constantly added to the lens and, along with other changes, cause the lens to grow stiffer and become less able to change its shape. Beyond the age of 40–50 years, the lens provides little accommodative power to the eye, a condition called presbyopia: Greek *presbys* (an old man) + *opia*.

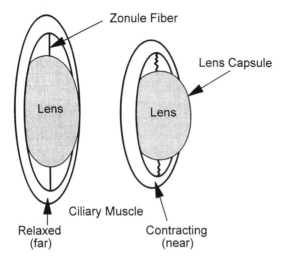

Figure 3.17. Ciliary muscle action during accommodation in primates. When the ciliary muscle contracts during accommodation for near objects, its sphincter-like action decreases the distance between the origin of the zonule fibers and the lens capsule, reducing the tension on the latter and allowing elastic forces within the lens to increase its curvature and optical power. This schematic diagram illustrates the effect on only two of the many zonule fibers attached to the equator of the lens.

When an object is brought toward the face, three events combine to permit the object to remain in sharp focus on the foveas of the two eyes. This near response comprises lens accommodation (increasing its optical power), pupillary constriction (increasing the depth of field), and inward movement of the visual axes (adduction) of both eyes. The afferent limb of the near response involves the retina and its central projections. All of the motor elements of the response are mediated by the oculomotor nerve or third cranial nerve.

Other Solutions to the Problem of Accommodation

The corneas of aquatic species generally contribute little to image formation, because the index of refraction of water is essentially the same as that of the aqueous humor, eliminating any significant net refraction by the parallel surfaces of the cornea. Consequently, it is left to the lens to form images on the retina and provide any active accommodative capacity available to the animal. The lenses of many fish are almost perfectly spherical, giving them great optical power, but potentially introducing a large

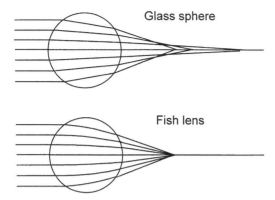

Figure 3.18. Comparison of refraction by a glass sphere and a fish lens. Spherical aberration is reduced and optical power increased by allowing the refractive index of the lens to be higher in the center than at the periphery. Light rays are refracted throughout the lens, rather than just at its surfaces.

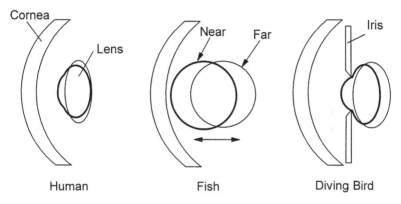

Figure 3.19. Accommodative strategies in humans, fish, and diving birds. Heavy outlines represent lens profiles during accommodation for near objects.

amount of spherical aberration. This problem has been solved by the development of lens material that decreases in refractive index from the center to the periphery (Figure 3.18). Light is bent not only at the surface of such a lens but also continuously as it traverses the lens. Image-forming devices based on this principle are found in invertebrates as well and have evolved many times.

To adjust the eye for different viewing distances, many fish can move the lens by means of intraocular muscles. Depending on the species, the active movement may be in the plane of the pupil or along its axis, toward or away from the retina (Figure 3.19). Snakes and adult amphibians also can move the lens to accommodate, either by muscles acting directly on the structures supporting the lens or by increasing intraocular pressure.

As already described for the human eye, a general accommodative strategy of vertebrates is to vary the optical power of the lens by changing its shape. Many birds and some reptiles (turtles and lizards) do this through the action of their ciliary and iris sphincter muscles, which are striated, rather than smooth like those of their mammalian counterparts. Although strategies vary from one species to another, the general pattern is for the ciliary muscle to compress the lens at its equator, moving the anterior surface forward and steepening its curvature. The powerful sphincter of the iris increases the rigidity of this structure and may even pinch the anterior part of the lens, contributing to its increased curvature (Figure 3.19). These muscular actions are aided by cartilaginous or bony plates that strengthen the sclera near its junction with the cornea.

Diving birds, such as cormorants and ducks, are able to increase the refractive power of their eyes 70–80 D by means of such mechanisms, allowing the eyes to form useful images in air and under water. Less is known about the accommodative mechanisms of amphibious mammals such as otters and seals, although the former have been reported to possess mechanisms like those of birds, and the latter to have spherical lenses like fish.

Further Reading

Fernald, R. D. (1988). Aquatic adaptations in fish eyes. In *Sensory Biology of Aquatic Animals*. ed. J. Atema, R. R. Fay, A. N. Popper, and W. N. Tavolga, pp. 435–66. Berlin: Springer-Verlag.

Jenkins, F. A., and White, H. E. (1957). *Fundamentals of Optics*. New York: McGraw-Hill.

Land, M. F. (1981). Optics and vision in invertebrates. In *Handbook of Sensory Physiology*, vol. 7, part 6B, ed. H. Autrum, pp. 471–592. Berlin: Springer-Verlag.

Land, M. F., and Fernald, R. D. (1992). The evolution of eyes. *Annual Review of Neuroscience* 15:1–30.

Nicol, J. A. C. (1989). *The Eyes of Fishes*. Oxford: Clarendon Press.

Sivak, J. G. (1980). Accommodation in vertebrates: a contemporary survey. *Current Topics in Eye Research* 3:281–330.

Sivak, J. G., Hildebrand, T., and Lebert, C. (1985). Magnitude and rate of accommodation in diving and nondiving birds. *Vision Research* 25:925–33.

Southall, J. P. C. (1964). *Mirrors, Prisms and Lenses*. New York: Dover.

CHAPTER 4

CENTRAL VISUAL PATHWAYS

This chapter provides an overview of the projections from the retina to the brain in vertebrates and reviews the key terms used in describing the pathway. The major components of the pathway and their functions are examined in greater detail in subsequent chapters.

The Visual Fields

The central projections of the two eyes map the visible world onto the brain. To understand this process, it is important to know how the visual field of each eye is described and how the projections from the two eyes are combined in the central pathways. The retina of each eye is conventionally divided into nasal and temporal parts, on the basis of proximity to the nose or temporal bone, respectively. Similarly, the visual field of each eye is divided into nasal and temporal parts, and because of the inversion of the retinal image by the eye's optics, the nasal visual field is imaged on the temporal retina, and the temporal field on the nasal retina. Figure 4.1 schematizes the projections of the visual fields in an animal whose eyes are located at the sides of its head. In such lateral-eyed animals, the axons from one retina generally cross completely in the optic chiasm, so that the input from that eye is directed at the contralateral hemisphere of the brain.

Figure 4.2 illustrates diagrammatically the monocular visual fields as

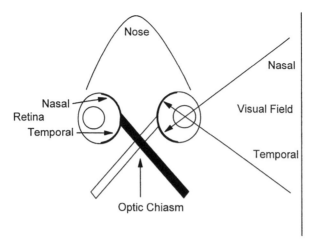

Figure 4.1. The visual fields as viewed by an animal with eyes located laterally on the sides of its head.

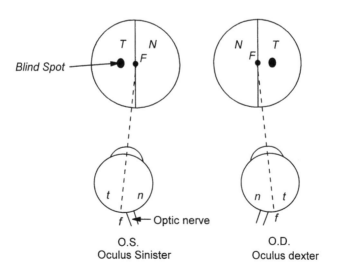

Figure 4.2. Schematic representation of the monocular visual fields of humans. T, temporal field; N, nasal field; F, fixation point; n, nasal retina; t, temporal retina; f, fovea. The dashed line is the visual axis or line of sight. By convention, the visual fields are always drawn as they appear to the observer.

they would appear to a frontal-eyed human observer, left eye (oculus sinister, O.S.) on the left, right eye (oculus dexter, O.D.) on the right. For each eye there are nasal and temporal visual fields defined with respect to the fixation point and the observer's nose and temple. Similarly, each retina has nasal and temporal sides, defined with respect to its fovea. The optic disc, where the ganglion cells' axons interrupt the retina to enter the optic nerve, is in the nasal retina and causes a blind spot in the temporal visual field. The fields illustrated in Figure 4.2 are highly schematic. In humans the temporal fields are more extensive than the nasal fields, and the borders of the fields are not perfectly circular.

Figure 4.3 schematizes the projection of the binocular visual field when a person's two eyes are open and are fixating a point F. The right hemifield (black) is imaged on both the nasal retina of the right eye and the temporal retina of the left eye, and vice versa for the left hemifield. Only the nasal retinal fibers decussate at the optic chiasm, and this, together with the optical inversion of the retinal image, causes the right and left visual hemifields to be "seen" respectively by the left and right (i.e., contralateral) hemispheres of the brain. Note also that the optic nerve contains axons from only one eye, whereas the optic chiasm and optic tract contain fibers from both eyes. At the extreme periphery of the visual field there is a zone seen only by the eye on that side (i.e., by the nasal retina of the ipsilateral eye). This area is sometimes called the monocular crescent or monocular segment.

In the following sections we consider the principal structures in the brain that receive direct input from the retina. Conscious visual perception in primates depends critically on the pathway from the retina to the lateral geniculate nucleus (LGN) of the thalamus and thence to the cerebral cortex (Figure 4.4). Retinal fibers also project to the superior colliculus of the midbrain, the pretectum, a complex of brain-stem nuclei called the accessory optic system, and the hypothalamus.

The Retino-geniculo-cortical Projection

In mammals, many axons in the optic tract project to the lateral geniculate nucleus of the thalamus, where they synapse on neurons in distinct dorsal and ventral components of this complex. The principal or relay neurons of the dorsal lateral geniculate send their axons to a region of the occipital cortex called, variously, the striate cortex, Brodmann's area 17, calcarine cortex, primary visual cortex, or V1 (Figures 4.4 and 4.5). The origins of these terms are discussed in Chapter 8. In some species, the cortical targets of axons from the lateral geniculate nucleus include Brodmann's areas 18 and 19 and still other regions of extrastriate cortex.

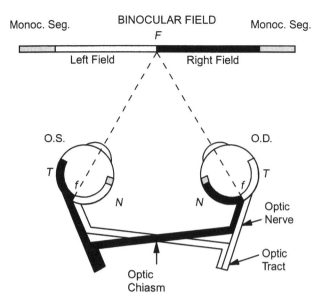

Figure 4.3. Schematic representation of the projection of the binocular visual field.
F, fixation point; *f*, fovea; *N*, nasal; *T*, temporal. Dashed line is the visual axis or
line of sight.

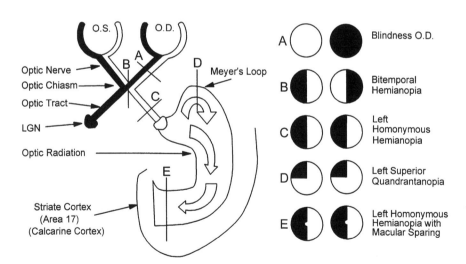

Figure 4.4. Visual-field defects due to lesions at different points in the retino-
geniculo-striate pathway. Interruption of the pathway at points A–E on the left
results in the corresponding visual-field defects on the right. LGN, lateral geniculate nucleus.

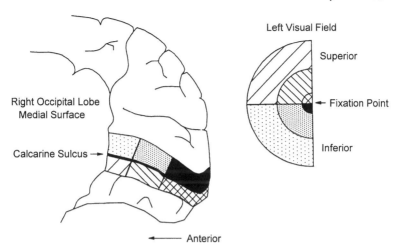

Figure 4.5. Retinotopy in the projection from the left visual field to the right occipital lobe.

The paths taken by fibers representing various parts of the visual field can best be appreciated by examining the effects of lesions in the visual pathway. Damage to the neurons of the visual pathway causes a "hole" in the visual field called a scotoma (plural, scotomata). This may be a completely blind area (dense scotoma) or one with reduced vision (partial or incomplete scotoma). The normal blind spot is, in effect, a scotoma, but it is not usually referred to as such. The term is generally reserved for pathological defects in the visual field. When a visual field defect occurs in only one eye, it is usually due to damage to the retina or the optic nerve (Figure 4.4, lesion A). Transection of the optic chiasm in the midline interrupts fibers crossing from the nasal retinas that carry information from the temporal visual fields. The resulting deficit is called a bitemporal hemianopia, because there is absence of vision in the temporal half-field of each eye (lesion B).

Interruption of the visual pathway behind the chiasm produces scotomata affecting the same hemifield of each eye. Thus, lesion C in Figure 4.4 produces a left homonymous hemianopia ("homonymous" means "same name" and refers to the fact that in this case the left hemifield of each eye is affected). Above the lateral geniculate nucleus the fibers in the optic radiation spread out, so a circumscribed lesion is not likely to interrupt all of them. Fibers representing the upper visual field occupy the lower part of the optic radiation and dip into the temporal lobe in what is called Meyer's loop. Damage here causes a superior quadrantanopia (lesion D in Figure 4.4). Damage higher in the pathway, and close to the visual cortex, often spares the representation of the central part of the visual field corresponding to the macular area of the retina, which contains the fovea (lesion E in Figure 4.4). This macular sparing is probably due to a number of factors. Because the representation of the macular area is very large in the cortex, parts of it are more likely to survive an injury than are regions with smaller representations. The macular area may also be supplied by more than one cerebral artery and thus be spared damage due to vascular disease. Other causes have been suggested, but evidence for them is scanty.

The retinal projection via the lateral geniculate nucleus to the striate cortex of the occipital lobe preserves near-neighbor relationships, so adjacent points in the contralateral visual field are represented at adjacent cortical points. In this retinotopic map, the superior half of the visual field is represented ventrally, and the inferior half dorsally, with respect to the calcarine sulcus. The fovea is represented on the most posterior aspect of the calcarine cortex at the occipital pole (Figure 4.5).

The central part of the visual field receives a disproportionately large representation in the striate cortex (Figure 4.5). This variable expansion of the representation of visual space can be expressed quantitatively in terms of a magnification factor, defined as the number of linear millimeters in the cortex (or other projection area) allotted to a given linear angle of visual space. Thus, one degree of visual angle might occupy 6 mm of cortex near the foveal representation (magnification factor = 6 mm/degree) and only 1 mm in peripheral parts of the map. Magnification can also be defined in terms of the area of cortex representing a degree of solid angle in visual space and expressed as square millimeters per degree squared. The notion of magnification factor plays a prominent role in a later discussion of spatial analysis by the visual system.

The reasons why central regions of the retina are accorded expanded representation in the visual cortex are not entirely understood, but one factor is that proportionately greater numbers of ganglion cells relay signals from this region than from equivalent areas in the peripheral retina. If the terminals of all retinal ganglion cells were allotted about the same amount of space in the lateral geniculate nucleus, the central part of the field would claim the most territory simply because it is represented by the largest number of cells. The projection from lateral geniculate to cortex would preserve this pattern. Quantitative studies, in fact, have shown that areal magnification factors in the striate cortex of the macaque are more or less proportional to the numbers of retinal ganglion cells representing the corresponding parts of the visual field (Figure 4.6), although there is evidence that the foveal representation

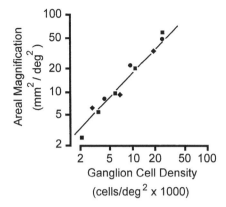

Figure 4.6. Proportionality of areal magnification in the striate cortex and retinal ganglion cell density in the macaque monkey. Ganglion cell density takes into account cells from both eyes contributing to the retino-geniculo-striate system on one side. (Reprinted from H. Wässle, U. Grünert, J. Rohrenbeck, and B. B. Boycott: Retinal ganglion cell density and cortical magnification factor in the primate. *Vision Research* 30:1897–911. Copyright 1990, with kind permission from Elsevier Science, Ltd., The Boulevard, Langford Lane, Kidlington OX5 1GB, United Kingdom.)

may be magnified to a greater degree in central maps than can be accounted for solely on the basis of the distribution of retinal ganglion cells.

The Retino-tectal or Retino-collicular Projection

The superior colliculus, part of the tectum of the midbrain, receives a major input from the retina through the retino-tectal projection (Figure 4.7), which generates a retinotopic map of the contralateral visual field, and in some animals the ipsilateral as well. This structure is involved in a variety of functions, including the control of visual orienting reflexes. In primates, many of its functions have been assumed by the retino-geniculo-cortical system, but its circuitry plays an essential role in the visually guided behavior of other animals. Although the superior colliculus does not provide a direct route from the retina to the visual cortex, a projection does exist via certain nuclei of the thalamus, including the lateral posterior and pulvinar nuclei. The functions of this extrageniculate pathway to the cerebral cortex are not understood.

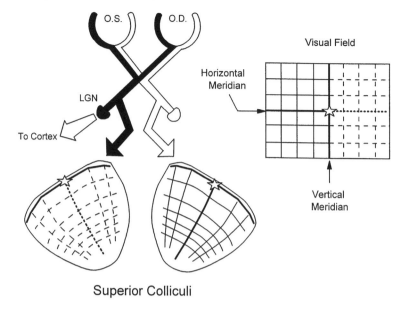

Figure 4.7. Projection of the visual field (right) to the superior colliculi (left). The coordinate systems illustrate a quantitative retinotopic mapping. The vertical and horizontal meridians of the visual field cross at the fixation point (star), which is represented at the rostral edge of both superior colliculi.

The Retino-pretectal Projection

The retina also projects to the pretectum, a region just rostral to the superior colliculus that comprises several distinct nuclei with different output projections and functions. This complex of nuclei controls, among other things, certain automatic movements of the eyes and the response of the pupil to light. The pathway of the pupillary light reflex is diagrammed in Figure 4.8. Note that the afferent fibers from each eye project to both pretectal areas, where they synapse. Fibers from each pretectal area project bilaterally to the Edinger-Westphal nuclei, collections of preganglionic parasympathetic neurons adjacent to the nuclei of the oculomotor nerves. From the Edinger-Westphal nucleus, axons travel via the oculomotor nerve to the orbit, where they synapse in the ciliary ganglion. The cholinergic postganglionic fibers proceed to the eye over ciliary nerves. Because of the bilateral connections in this circuitry, illumination of one eye causes pupillary constriction in that eye (direct response) and in the opposite eye (consensual response). The redundancy in the projection makes it difficult to interrupt this reflex.

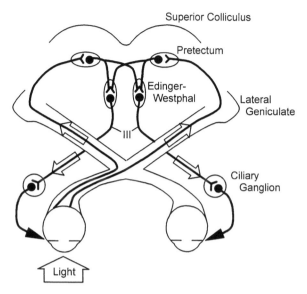

Figure 4.8. Pathway of the pupillary light reflex via the pretectum, Edinger-Westphal nucleus, and ciliary ganglion. Observe that light entering one eye results in bilateral activation of the pretectal nuclei, each of which activates both Edinger-Westphal nuclei. Thus, illumination of one retina causes both ipsilateral pupillary constriction (the direct reflex) and contralateral constriction (the consensual reflex). Because of this redundancy, post-chiasmatic lesions of the visual pathway rarely interrupt the reflex.

The Accessory Optic System

The mammalian retina projects directly to several small nuclei located bilaterally along the ventral and lateral surfaces of the midbrain. Whereas mammals generally have three such accessory optic nuclei on each side, nonmammals usually have only one. Cells in these nuclei project to brainstem regions involved in the generation of eye movements and, together with nuclei of the pretectal area, are important in controlling reflex movements of the eyes that help stabilize the direction of gaze.

The Retino-hypothalamic Projection

Axons of certain retinal ganglion cells exit the optic chiasm just beneath the hypothalamus and terminate in the suprachiasmatic nucleus. This projection is thought to be important in the synchronization of diurnal biological rhythms with the day–night cycle.

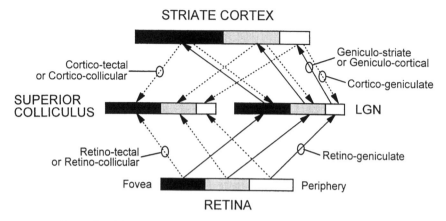

Figure 4.9. Schematic representation of the retino-geniculo-striate and retino-tectal projections and the return projections from the visual cortex.

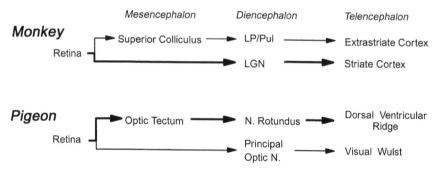

Figure 4.10. Comparison of major visual pathways in monkey and pigeon. LP/Pul, lateral posterior and pulvinar nuclei; LGN, lateral geniculate nucleus, pars dorsalis. The relative strengths of the projections are indicated by the thickness of the arrows.

Descending Cortical Projections

The visual cortex not only receives visual information from the lateral geniculate nucleus but also sends a reciprocal projection back to that nucleus, the cortico-geniculate projection. The superior colliculus is also a major target of corticofugal axons from the visual cortex, via the cortico-tectal or cortico-collicular projection. The cortico-tectal and cortico-geniculate projections are organized retinotopically. Figure 4.9 presents a schematic summary of the main pathways discussed here and also

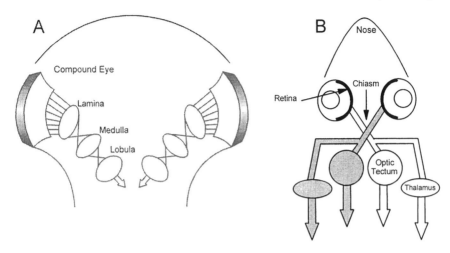

Figure 4.11. Comparison of central visual projections in a fly (A) and a vertebrate with lateral eyes (B).

illustrates the differential magnifications of the visual field in these projections.

Central Pathways in Nonmammalian Vertebrates and Invertebrates

The central visual pathways in nonmammalian vertebrates differ in important ways from those of mammals. Although the retina does project to nuclei in the thalamus and thence to telencephalic areas, its most prominent targets are the optic tectum of the midbrain and various other subcortical areas. The optic tectum, which is homologous to the mammalian superior colliculus, in turn projects to a variety of targets, including thalamic nuclei that project to the telencephalon. Telencephalic architecture in mammals differs significantly from that in other vertebrates, resulting in considerable variation in circuitry and nomenclature. The diagrams of Figure 4.10 compare the main ascending pathways in monkey and pigeon. Whereas the major projection in the monkey is to the striate cortex via the lateral geniculate nucleus, that in the pigeon is to the dorsal ventricular ridge of the telencephalon via the optic tectum of the midbrain and the nucleus rotundus of the thalamus.

In some nonmammalian species, primarily reptiles, birds, and fish, centrifugal fibers from the brain carry information back to the retina. These projections arise from brain-stem nuclei in some species and from the telencephalon in others and may modulate the responsiveness of retinal amacrine and ganglion cells. The presence of such centrifugal systems in mammals is still a matter of controversy.

The central visual pathways of invertebrates differ greatly from the vertebrate pattern (Figure 4.11) and vary significantly among invertebrate species. In an advanced invertebrate system, such as that of the fly, neural signals from one compound eye are transmitted centrally through a chain of ganglia located on the same side of the head (Figure 4.11A). Complex circuitry in these ganglia transforms the signals before sending them on to the rest of the nervous system.

Further Reading

Carpenter, M. B. (1976). *Human Neuroanatomy*, 7th ed. Baltimore: Williams & Wilkins.

Douglas, R. H., and Djamgoz, M. B. A. (eds.) (1990). *The Visual System of Fish*. London: Chapman & Hall.

Harrington, D. O. (1981). *The Visual Fields*, 5th ed. St. Louis: Mosby.

Polyak, S. (1957). *The Vertebrate Visual System*. University of Chicago Press.

Shimizu, T., and Karten, H. J. (1991). Central visual pathways in reptiles and birds: evolution of the visual system. In *Vision and Visual Dysfunction. Vol. 2: Evolution of the Visual System*, ed. J. R. Cronly-Dillon and R. L. Gregory, pp. 421–41. Boca Raton: CRC Press.

Uchiyama, H. (1989). Centrifugal pathways to the retina: influence of the optic tectum. *Visual Neuroscience* 3:183–206.

PART II

NEURAL MECHANISMS

CHAPTER 5

PHOTORECEPTORS AND PHOTORECEPTION

Photoreceptor Anatomy

Figure 5.1 illustrates the basic components of vertebrate photoreceptors. The outer segment is a specialized cilium containing large numbers of disc-like expansions of the cell membrane. The outer segment is connected by the ciliary stalk to the inner segment, a structure that acts as a light pipe, guiding incident photons to the light-sensitive pigments. The inner segment also contains large numbers of mitochondria that house part of the biochemical machinery required to meet the metabolic needs of the photoreceptor. An axon-like process of variable length connects the cell body to the synaptic terminal, where contact is made with the next elements of the visual pathway. Vertebrate retinas generally possess two types of photoreceptors, called rods and cones, after the shapes of their outer segments. The receptor schematized in Figure 5.1 is a rod. As the name implies, the outer segments of cones taper toward the tip.

The electron micrograph of a rhesus monkey's cone in Figure 5.2 shows the ciliary stalk and part of the outer segment with its stack of discs, including discs newly forming near the ciliary stalk (arrow). The photopigments, which absorb light and initiate the visual process, form a major structural element in these membranous discs. Also visible in the figure are the mitochondria packing the inner segment. In cones, the disc membranes are continuous over the surface of the outer segment and present

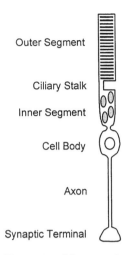

Outer Segment

Ciliary Stalk

Inner Segment

Cell Body

Axon

Synaptic Terminal

Figure 5.1. Schematic diagram of vertebrate photoreceptor. The outer segment contains membranous discs (black lines), and the inner segment contains mitochondria (stippled ovals).

one face to the extracellular space. Rods differ in that the newly formed discs pinch off from the plasma membrane and are stacked like poker chips inside the more or less cylindrical outer segment.

Phototransduction in the Rod

When an electrode is placed near an isolated photoreceptor that is shielded from light, it registers the presence of a large current, the dark current, that flows into the outer segment, through the cell, and out of the inner segment, completing the circuit in the extracellular fluid (Figure 5.3A). The greater part of the current entering the outer segment is carried by sodium ions (Na^+), and the remainder by calcium ions (Ca^{2+}) and some magnesium ions (Mg^{2+}). Current leaving the photoreceptor's inner segment is carried largely by potassium ions (K^+). A membrane-bound pump, driven by metabolic energy, exchanges extracellular K^+ for intracellular Na^+ and maintains the ionic concentration gradients needed to sustain the dark current. Calcium entering the outer segment is removed by an exchanger or countertransporter that transfers four Na^+ into the cell and expels one Ca^{2+} and one K^+.

In the dark, the relatively large influx of Na^+ drives the membrane potential of the photoreceptor toward the sodium equilibrium potential and keeps the membrane relatively depolarized. As in other neurons, this

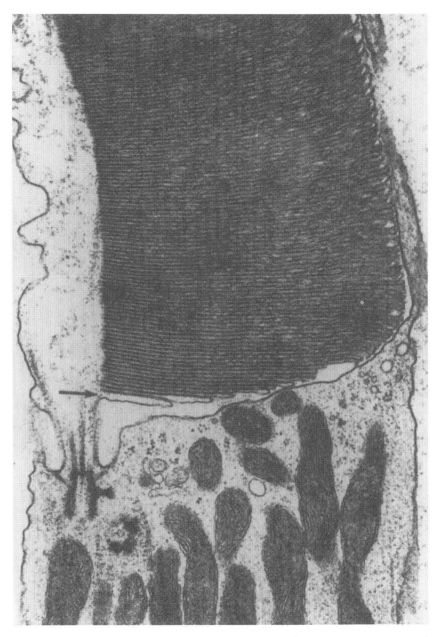

Figure 5.2. Electron micrograph of the transition from inner to outer segment in a rhesus monkey's cone. The arrow just above the ciliary stalk points to a newly forming disc. Numerous mitochondria are visible just below the stalk in the inner segment. (Reprinted from R. H. Steinberg, S. K. Fisher, and D. H. Anderson: Disc morphogenesis in vertebrate photoreceptors. *Journal of Comparative Neurology* 190:501–18. Copyright 1980, by permission of Wiley-Liss, Inc., a subsidiary of John Wiley & Sons.)

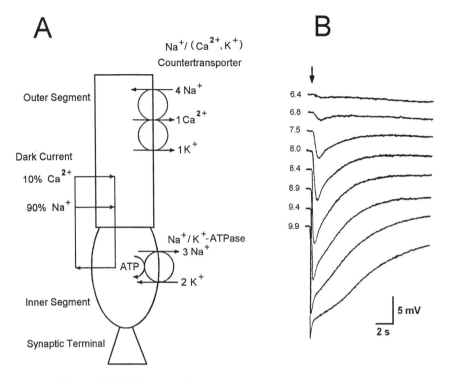

Figure 5.3. (A) Diagram of rod photoreceptor showing dark-current path and ion transporters and pumps. (Reprinted from G. L. Fain and H. R. Matthews: Calcium and the mechanism of light adaptation in vertebrate photoreceptors. *Trends in Neurosciences* 13:378–84, 1990, with permission of Elsevier Trends Journals.) (B) Intracellular recordings from a toad rod showing hyperpolarizing responses to a light flash (arrow). Numbers to left show stimulus intensity in units of log quanta per square millimeter per flash. (Reprinted from G. L. Fain, G. H. Gold, and J. E. Dowling: Receptor coupling in the toad retina. *Cold Spring Harbor Symposium on Quantitative Biology* 40:547–61, 1975, with permission of the Cold Spring Harbor Laboratory.)

depolarization leads to release of neurotransmitter at the receptor terminal, so vertebrate photoreceptors release their transmitter at maximal rates in the dark. Exposure of the photoreceptor to light causes the cation channels of the outer segment to close, with the result that the membrane potential becomes relatively hyperpolarized as it moves toward the potassium equilibrium potential (Figure 5.3B). In short, light hyperpolarizes the vertebrate photoreceptor and decreases the release of transmitter from the receptor terminal. Only about 1% of the cation channels are open in darkness, and it is this small fraction of the existing channels that are switched between the open and closed states by light. Under normal circumstances, the photoreceptors do not generate action potentials.

The effect of light on the dark current is spatially restricted. If a narrow beam is focused on a short span of the outer segment, only the current entering that span is reduced. A key question, then, is how the absorption of light by a molecule of photopigment affects the cation channels in the nearby membrane. The first step in this process is a transformation of the photopigment molecule itself, as described next.

Photopigments

As noted in Chapter 1, all of the photosensitive pigments employed by the eyes of animals are composed of a form of vitamin A, the chromophore, and a membrane-bound protein called an opsin. The structures of vitamin A and two of its aldehydes are illustrated in Figure 5.4. Figure 5.5 shows the chromophore associated with the opsin. When the 11-*cis* isomer of retinaldehyde (11-*cis* retinal) absorbs a single photon, it is isomerized to the all-*trans* form, and this change in shape of the chromophore converts the opsin to an activated state, triggering subsequent events in the transduction process, as discussed in detail later. After observing that illumination of receptor pigments caused them to become lighter in color, early investigators called the process bleaching, a term still used to refer to these early stages of phototransduction.

Rhodopsin, composed of 11-*cis* retinaldehyde and a specific opsin, is the photopigment of the vertebrate rod photoreceptor. The spectral sensitivity of human rhodopsin is virtually identical to that of the dark-adapted eye measured psychophysically, indicating that rhodopsin is in fact the photopigment responsible for vision at these low light levels. The cone photopigments also contain 11-*cis* retinaldehyde, but the opsins differ from that of rhodopsin. Related forms are also present in invertebrates and some unicellular organisms.

The Enzymatic Cascade

In 1942, S. Hecht, S. Shlaer, and M. H. Pirenne demonstrated that simultaneous absorptions of about five to seven light quanta in a patch of rods could reliably produce a detectable sensation of light in humans. Their analysis also showed that when these very faint flashes were detected, the probability that any single rod had absorbed two quanta of light was disappearingly small. From this they concluded that a behaviorally detectable signal was generated when one rhodopsin molecule was isomerized in each of a few rods. Electrical recordings from the eye of the horseshoe

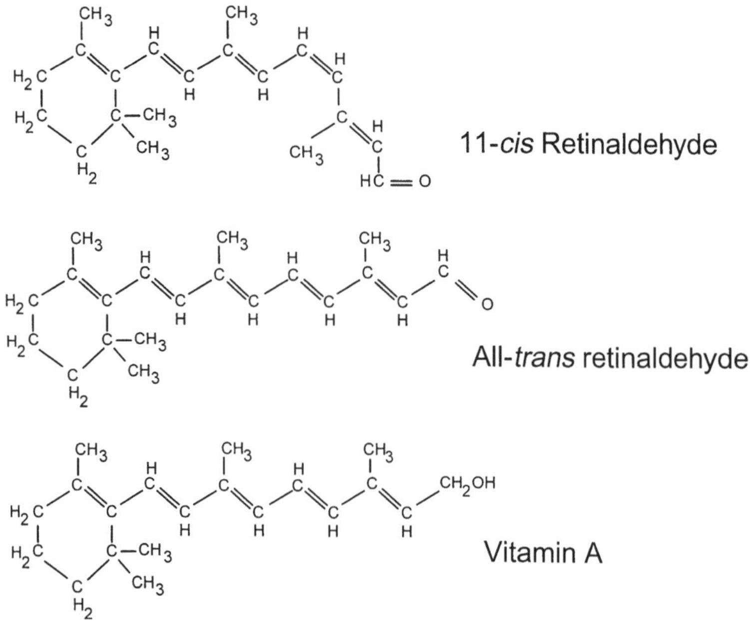

Figure 5.4. Chemical structures of vitamin A and its 11-*cis* and all-*trans* aldehydes. Absorption of a quantum of light isomerizes ll-*cis* retinal to the all-*trans* form.

crab later revealed that absorption of a single quantum could produce an electrical event requiring far more energy than that involved in the isomerization of a single molecule of rhodopsin. This led to the search for a process of amplification by which the isomerization of the photopigment could trigger other events of the appropriate magnitude.

Intracellular recordings and recordings from small patches of vertebrate photoreceptor membrane have established that the light-sensitive cation channels of the outer segments are kept open by cytoplasmic cGMP (cyclic guanosine monophosphate). Light must somehow reduce the levels of cGMP to affect the dark current and the membrane potential of the receptor. The major events leading to this reduction have now been identified and are illustrated schematically in Figure 5.6. The critical steps are these:

1. Photoactivated rhodopsin (R*) converts the protein transducin (T) to its active form (T*).
2. T* activates phosphodiesterase (PDE → PDE*).
3. PDE* converts cGMP to GMP.
4. Reduction of cGMP concentration closes the cation channels and reduces the inward flow of positive ions, hyperpolarizing the photoreceptor and slowing transmitter release.

Cytoplasmic
Surface

Lipid Bilayer

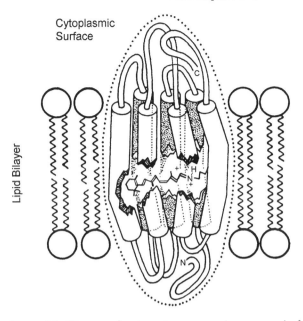

Figure 5.5. Diagram of a photopigment complex composed of a molecule of ret-inaldehyde nestled within the seven membrane-spanning elements of the opsin. The photopigment is an integral part of the cell membrane and is surrounded by the lipid bilayer. (Adapted from E. A. Dratz and P. A. Hargrave: The structure of rhodopsin and the rod outer segment disk membrane. *Trends in Biochemical Sciences* 8:128–31, 1983, with permission of Elsevier Trends Journals.)

Activated rhodopsin (R*) may convert several thousand transducins to the active form, and activated phosphodiesterase (PDE*) decyclizes many cGMP molecules. Isomerization of one rhodopsin molecule in the outer segment decreases the dark current by about 3%, which represents an enormous amplification of the energy contributed by the quantum of light to the rhodopsin molecule.

Recovery of Receptor Sensitivity

The photoreceptors must reliably signal the occurrence of different photic events over time, which means that the effects of a single exposure to light must be short-lived. The processes ensuring this do so by limiting the lifetimes of the active forms of rhodopsin, transducin, and phosphodiesterase, and also by restoring intracellular levels of cGMP. These events proceed in parallel:

Photoreceptor Outer Segment

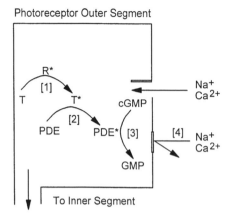

Figure 5.6. Schematic diagram of the enzymatic cascade that results in closure of cation channels in the outer segment. Numbers in brackets correspond to the steps described in the text. (Reproduced with permission of the Grass Instrument Company.)

1. Activated rhodopsin is rapidly inactivated by a sequence of phosphorylations and binding by a protein called arrestin. The inactivated photopigment undergoes further internal transformations and finally dissociates into the opsin and the chromophore in its all-*trans* form. The opsin remains associated with the disc membrane, and the all-*trans* retinal is converted to its alcohol form (retinol or vitamin A), transported to the pigment epithelium, and re-isomerized to 11-*cis* retinol. This molecule is then returned to the photoreceptor outer segment, oxidized, and recombined with opsin. If the retina is isolated from the pigment epithelium, it does not recover its sensitivity after bleaching.
2. Activated transducin has the capacity to inactivate itself. This auto-inactivation proceeds slowly enough for the activated transducin to play its role in the enzymatic cascade.
3. cGMP is constantly formed from cytoplasmic GMP by the enzyme guanylate cyclase. Exposure of the photoreceptor to light results in an increase in the activity of this enzyme, accelerating the conversion of GMP to cGMP. This process has an effect opposite to that of activated phosphodiesterase and therefore represents a kind of negative feedback. The activity of guanylate cyclase is controlled by intracellular Ca^{2+} concentration, which is momentarily reduced by light as the outer segment's cation channels close and calcium influx drops.

It should be evident at this point that the response of the photoreceptor to light is governed by a complex, interacting network of biochemical and biophysical processes. A major focus of retinal research is to characterize these interactions thoroughly and to develop a detailed, quantitative model of the process.

The Na^+/K^+ Pump and Oxygen Consumption in Photoreceptors

The cationic pump operating in the inner segment to maintain normal concentration gradients of Na^+ and K^+ consumes large amounts of metabolic energy in the form of adenosine triphosphate (ATP). The dark current has been estimated to turn over all the cations of the cell every 47 seconds and to consume 5×10^6 molecules of ATP per rod per second. Production of the ATP is carried out in the mitochondria, which are densely packed in the inner segment (Figures 5.1 and 5.2). Oxygen is consumed at so high a rate in this process that the extracellular oxygen tension falls from the high levels of choroidal blood to essentially zero near the inner segments.

Retinal hypoxia slows the Na^+/K^+ pump and results in depolarization of the photoreceptors. Even mild hypoxia, such as that experienced by passengers flying at high altitudes in commercial aircraft, is said to cause the cabin lights to appear dimmer than they do on the ground. The depolarization induced by hypoxia may explain why pressure on the sclera behind the retina produces a dark spot in the opposite visual field. By occluding the choroidal circulation, the pressure leads to a local depolarization of the photoreceptors that would normally be associated with a region of darkness in the visual field.

Outer-Segment Turnover and Renewal of Discs

The cycle of bleaching and regeneration of the photopigments occurs on a time scale of seconds and minutes. Another process slowly replaces the outer segments of the photoreceptors over the course of several days. By labeling newly synthesized proteins with radioactive amino acids, R. W. Young showed that the membranous discs formed near the ciliary bridge of a rod's outer segment (see arrow in Figure 5.2) migrate outward as new discs are formed and finally are shed from the tip and phagocytosed by the pigment epithelium (Figure 5.7).

In rats, shedding of rod discs occurs at about daybreak in a circadian rhythm and continues if the animal is kept in the dark. The shedding in goldfish is controlled by changes in illumination and is not under circadian control. Rods shed during periods of light, and cones in the dark. The outer segment of a human photoreceptor turns over completely in 9–13 days.

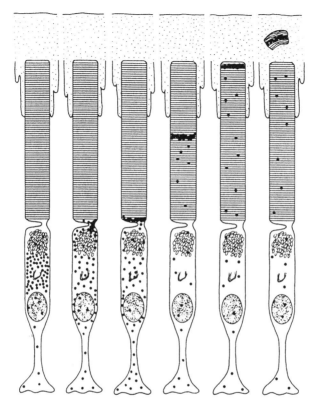

Figure 5.7. Renewal of outer-segment discs. Radioactive amino acids (black dots) injected on day 1 (left) appear in proteins at the base of the outer segment and move progressively toward the pigment epithelium, where they are shed after about 10 days. (Courtesy of Dr. R. W. Young. Reprinted from *Textbook of Medical Physiology*, 13th ed., ed. V. B. Mountcastle. St. Louis: Mosby. Copyright 1974, with permission of the C. V. Mosby Co.)

Photoreception in the Invertebrate Eye

Invertebrate photoreceptors differ from those of vertebrates in a number of important ways. In a compound eye, such as that of a crustacean (Figure 5.8), each ommatidium possesses its own optical elements and includes several photoreceptors that constitute the <u>retinula</u> (little retina). The part of the retinular cell corresponding functionally to the vertebrate outer segment is not a specialized cilium, but rather is formed of microvillar extensions of the plasma membrane, the <u>rhabdomer</u>. The rhabdomers collectively form the <u>rhabdom</u>. Although the retinular cells project indepen-

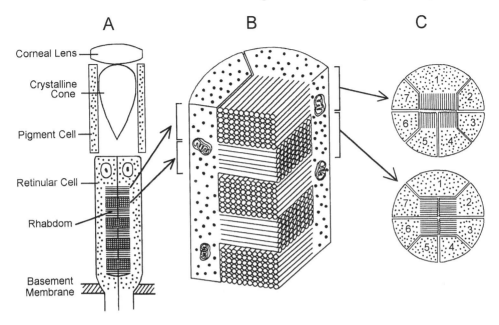

Figure 5.8. Schematic representation of an ommatidium in the compound eye of a crayfish. (A) Longitudinal section illustrating the image-forming apparatus of the corneal lens and crystalline cone, as well as two of the seven photoreceptor cells forming the neural component or retinula. The black dots represent pigment granules in pigment cells and retinular cells. The ommatidium is actually much longer than shown in this diagram. (B) A quarter segment of the ommatidium illustrating the microvillar contributions of two retinular cells to the rhabdom. (C) Schematic cross sections through the retinula showing that layers of the rhabdom are formed in alternation by rhabdomers from cells 1, 4, and 5 and from cells 2, 3, 6, and 7. (Adapted from E. Eguchi: Rhabdom structure and receptor potentials in single crayfish retinular cells. *Journal of Comparative and Cellular Physiology* 66:411–29, 1965, by permission of John Wiley & Sons, Inc.)

dently from the rhabdom, they may extend their rhabdomeric protrusions toward the central axis of the ommatidium, where they interlace (Figure 5.8B and C). The orthogonal arrangement of the rhabdomers and the constraints imposed by the membrane on the orientation of the photopigment may impart to the eye a sensitivity to the polarization angle of incident light. Not all compound eyes interdigitate the rhabdomers of a single ommatidium into a single, closed rhabdom. In the fly's eye, for instance, the rhabdom is open, and each retinular cell is selectively sensitive to light entering the ommatidium from a particular direction.

Phototransduction in invertebrates parallels that described earlier for the vertebrate rod, but with important differences. Activated rhodopsin, which is based on a vitamin A that differs slightly from its vertebrate counterpart, converts a specific transducin-like protein to its active form, which then activates a phospholipase C. This enzyme acts on a membrane phospholipid to produce inositol triphosphate (IP_3) and diacylglycerol, both intracellular second messengers. The IP_3 causes release of calcium ions stored in intracellular compartments, and this leads to the opening of cation channels in the photoreceptor membrane. Thus, as a rule, invertebrate photoreceptors are depolarized by light, although there are exceptions. An additional difference is that the chromophore and the opsin do not dissociate after absorption of light, the bleached rhodopsin being re-isomerized by subsequent quantal absorptions.

Further Reading

Baylor, D. A. (1987). Photoreceptor signals and vision. *Investigative Ophthalmology and Visual Science* 28:34–49.

Detwiler, P. B., and Gray-Keller, M. P. (1992). Some unresolved issues in the physiology and biochemistry of phototransduction. *Current Opinion in Neurobiology* 2:433–8.

Hamdorf, K. (1979). The physiology of invertebrate visual pigments. In *Handbook of Sensory Physiology*, vol. 7, part 6A, ed. H. Autrum, pp. 145–224. Berlin: Springer-Verlag.

Hecht, S., Shlaer, S., and Pirenne, M. H. (1942). Energy, quanta, and vision. *Journal of General Physiology* 6:819–40.

Ranganathan, R., Harris, W. A., and Zuker, C. S. (1991). The molecular genetics of invertebrate phototransduction. *Trends in Neurosciences* 14:486–93.

Rodieck, R. W. (1973). *The Retina*. San Francisco: Freeman.

Schwartz, E. A. (1985). Phototransduction in vertebrate rods. *Annual Review of Neuroscience* 8:339–67.

Stryer, L. (1986). Cyclic GMP cascade of vision. *Annual Review of Neuroscience* 9: 87–120.

Wald, G. (1960). The distribution and evolution of visual systems. In *Comparative Biochemistry: A Comprehensive Treatise*, vol. 1, ed. M. Florkin and H. S. Mason, pp. 311–45. New York: Academic Press.

Yau, K.-W., and Baylor, D. A. (1989). Cyclic GMP-activated conductance in retinal photoreceptor cells. *Annual Review of Neuroscience* 12:289–328.

Young, R. W. (1976). Visual cells and the concept of renewal. *Investigative Ophthalmology* 15:700–25.

CHAPTER 6

RETINAL CIRCUITRY

Cell Types and Laminae of the Vertebrate Retina

The retina is a part of the brain that is displaced into the periphery during embryonic development (see Chapter 2). Because it is relatively accessible, retinal tissue provides a useful experimental model of brain circuitry. Some of the most significant advances in our understanding have come from studies of the retinas of cold-blooded vertebrates, which contain large neurons amenable to intracellular recording and staining. Mud puppies, turtles, frogs, and fish have been particularly rich sources of information. The cells of the mammalian retina are more difficult to study, but much work has been done in primates, cats, rabbits, and rats. Although some general patterns of organization have emerged, it is clear that no retina is exactly like any other, not even among mammals. This must be kept in mind when extrapolating from the wealth of comparative data to mammalian retinas, and particularly primate retinas.

The lamination of the retina is a guide to the locations of the various cell types and to the regions in which they make synaptic contacts. The somata or perikarya of the photoreceptors form the outer nuclear layer (Figure 6.1), and their inner and outer segments lie between this layer and the pigment epithelium. Axonal processes of the photoreceptors extend toward the outer plexiform layer, where they establish contacts with bipolar cells and horizontal cells. The somata of bipolar cells and horizontal

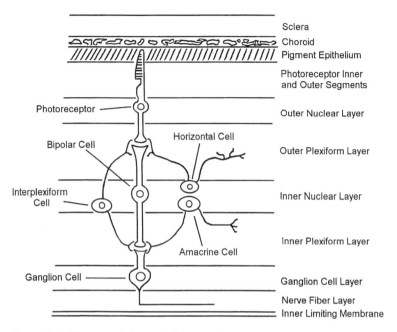

Figure 6.1. Diagram of the retinal layers showing the laminar locations of the principal types of cells. This diagram follows the anatomic convention of orienting the retina with the vitreous side down.

cells share the inner nuclear layer with those of amacrine cells, interplexiform cells, and Müller cells (glial cells unique to the retina). The inner plexiform layer is the site of synaptic interactions among amacrine, bipolar, and ganglion cells. In some species, interplexiform cells extend processes into both the inner and outer plexiform layers. Perikarya of the ganglion cells form the ganglion cell layer, and their axons proceed to the optic nerve via the nerve-fiber layer. The latter is separated from the vitreous by the inner limiting membrane, which represents the basement lamina of the optic vesicle.

The laminar distribution of cell types just described is the "standard" view of retinal organization, but recent studies indicate that the situation is considerably more complex. It has long been known that some ganglion cells have their perikarya in the inner nuclear layer rather than in the ganglion cell layer. In certain birds, these so-called displaced ganglion cells (Dogiel cells) have been found to project exclusively to nuclei of the accessory optic system in the brain stem. Because their apparently aberrant placement has a strong functional correlate, it is unlikely that their location is due to some error in development. It is now known that large numbers of neurons in the ganglion cell layer in rabbits and cats are actually amacrine cells that send their processes back into the inner plexiform layer. Traditionally such cells were called displaced amacrine cells, in the sense that they ended up in the "wrong" layer, but given their large numbers, it is unlikely that their displacement is accidental. A practical consequence of this is that one cannot estimate the number of ganglion cells simply by counting cell nuclei in the ganglion cell layer.

Synaptic Contacts of Mammalian Photoreceptors

In the outer plexiform layer, the synaptic terminals of rods and cones contact the processes of horizontal cells and bipolar cells whose somata lie in the inner nuclear layer. The terminals of cones are called pedicles because of their substantial size and large surface area. The smaller rod terminals are called spherules because of their more or less circular profiles. In mammals, a given bipolar cell makes contact with only rods or only cones, not with both. At one specialized junction, called a triad, the dendrite of a cone bipolar cell invaginates the cone pedicle and is flanked by two other invaginating processes that belong to horizontal cells (Figure 6.2, left). Opposite the three postsynaptic elements, the photoreceptor terminal contains an intracellular organelle called a synaptic ribbon, around which synaptic vesicles aggregate (arrowheads). The bipolar cell involved in this synapse is called an invaginating bipolar cell. Another type of contact occurring on the basal surface of cone pedicles does not press into the pedicle membrane but appears flat. The cells associated with these synapses are called flat bipolar cells (Figure 6.2, left, inset). Primates possess a subset of bipolar cells, called midget bipolar cells, that also have invaginating and flat synaptic morphologies. Midget bipolar cells are postsynaptic to a single cone in the central retina, where they provide the exclusive bipolar-cell input to a single midget ganglion cell. Midget ganglion cells occur throughout the primate retina, but receive convergent cone input in the periphery. Rod bipolar cells of mammals are all of the invaginating type and form the central elements in the triad junctions of the rod spherules (Figure 6.2, right).

Bipolar cells, like photoreceptors, respond to light with graded changes in membrane potential and do not generate action potentials. Light depolarizes invaginating bipolar cells, increasing the rate at which they release their transmitter (Figure 6.3). Thus the invaginating bipolar cell is often referred to as an on bipolar cell. In the flat bipolar cell, which is hyperpolarized by light (Figure 6.3), depolarization and increased transmitter release occur when the light goes off, so this cell is sometimes called an off bipolar cell.

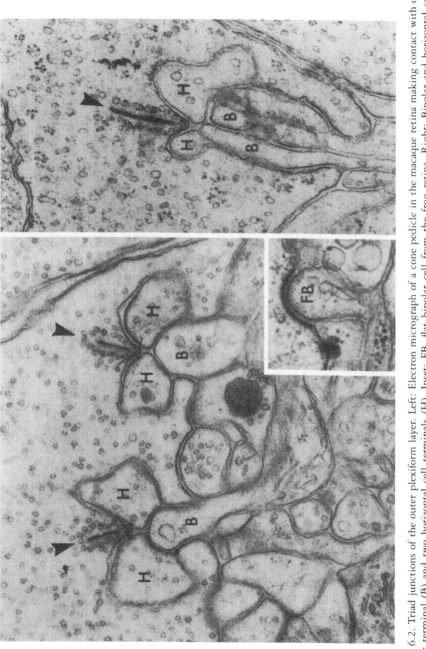

Figure 6.2. Triad junctions of the outer plexiform layer. Left: Electron micrograph of a cone pedicle in the macaque retina making contact with one bipolar terminal (B) and two horizontal cell terminals (H). Inset: FB, flat bipolar cell from the frog retina. Right: Bipolar and horizontal cells invaginating a rod spherule in the cat retina. Arrowheads point to synaptic ribbons in the presynaptic elements of each triad junction (Reprinted from J. E. Dowling: Organization of vertebrate retinas. *Investigative Ophthalmology and Visual Science* 9:655–80, 1970, with permission of the Association for Research in Vision and Ophthalmology.)

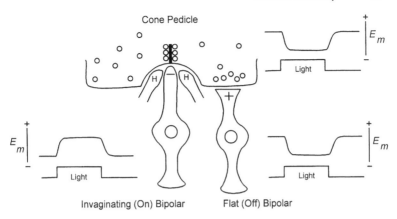

Figure 6.3. Schematic of the differential effects of light on the membrane potentials of a cone, an invaginating cone bipolar cell, and a flat cone bipolar cell. H, horizontal cell terminals in the triad junction. E_m, membrane potential.

Because the photoreceptor is hyperpolarized by light and decreases its transmitter output, it follows that the transmitter, probably the amino acid glutamate, inhibits the on bipolar cell and excites the off bipolar cell. The synapse between the cone and the on bipolar cell is said to be a sign-inverting synapse (indicated by the minus sign in the invaginating terminal in Figure 6.3), because hyperpolarization of the presynaptic cell causes depolarization of the postsynaptic cell. The contact between the photoreceptor and flat bipolar cell is sign-conserving (indicated by the plus sign in Figure 6.3). The mechanisms of action of the transmitter on the two types of bipolar cells are fundamentally different. Whereas the transmitter depolarizes the flat bipolar cell by opening ion channels directly, it acts on the invaginating bipolar cell through a protein related to transducin to reduce cGMP concentrations and close ion channels, a process analogous to that occurring in the photoreceptor when exposed to light. Rod bipolar cells are exclusively of the depolarizing or on type, which is consistent with the invaginating morphology of their dendritic terminals (Figure 6.2).

Thus, at the very first synapses in the visual pathway, separate systems are established to detect increments and decrements in retinal illumination. The on system and off system that emerge at this point initiate a fundamental coding strategy that persists throughout the rest of the visual system. A tool of great importance in studying these systems is the compound 2-amino-4-phosphonobutyrate (APB), an analogue of glutamate, which inhibits the on bipolar cell and disables the on system. APB binds to the glutamate receptors on the invaginating bipolar cells and continu-

ously hyperpolarizes them, so that they cannot liberate transmitter in response to an increment in illumination. An application of this agent in
the analysis of retinal circuitry will be described later.

Receptive Fields of Visual Cells

One of the most important concepts in sensory neurobiology is that of the
receptive field of a neuron. The receptive field of a visual cell is that region
of the retina (or the visual field) where a stimulus must be placed in order
to affect the cell. In its most general sense, "receptive field" can be defined
as the answer to this question: Here is a cell, where are the points that it
"sees"? In a typical experiment, the responses of a neuron are recorded
with a microelectrode while stimuli are projected on the retina, either
directly using specialized optics or indirectly by creating the stimuli on
an external surface and allowing the eye's own optics to form the retinal
image. The effect of light on any cell other than a photoreceptor is ultimately a function of that cell's connections to the photoreceptors, so the
cell's receptive field is, in some sense, an operational description of these
connections. The receptive field may include inhibitory as well as excitatory regions, and not all stimuli located within it may be effective. For
instance, a cell may require stimuli of a certain luminance configuration,
chromatic pattern, or movement direction. Each of these latter properties
qualifies the description of the receptive field, but does not modify its
fundamental attribute of location.

Receptive Fields of Bipolar Cells

The effect of light on a bipolar cell depends on whether it illuminates the
photoreceptors that contact the cell directly or those located in the surrounding area. It will be recalled that a bipolar cell does not generate
action potentials, the effect of light being to modulate its membrane potential up or down, depending on whether it is depolarized or hyperpolarized by the photoreceptor's transmitter. On bipolar cells are, by definition, depolarized by a centrally located spot of light, but are
hyperpolarized by light falling on adjacent photoreceptors (Figure 6.4).
These cells are depolarized when the peripheral spot is turned off, so their
receptive fields are said to comprise an on center and an off surround. The
converse is true for the off bipolar cells, which have off-center,
on-surround receptive fields.

The effects of illuminating the center of a bipolar cell's receptive field
are antagonistic to the effects of light in the surround. For instance, illumination of the off surround of an on-center bipolar cell reduces the

On-Center Bipolar

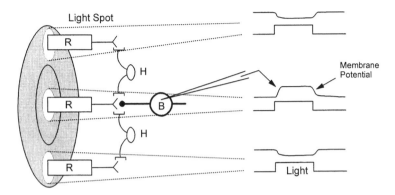

Receptive Field

Figure 6.4. Receptive field of an on-center bipolar cell. B, bipolar cell; H, horizontal cell; R, receptor. Small light spots projected on the retina cause depolarization when they illuminate receptors contacting the bipolar cell directly. Horizontal cells appear to mediate the hyperpolarizing effects of surround stimulation.

depolarizing response to illumination of the center. In some retinas, illumination of the receptive field's surround does not produce a direct change in membrane potential, but still counteracts or antagonizes responses evoked by simultaneous stimulation of the center. This phenomenon is often referred to as lateral inhibition, and it plays an important role in processing the retinal image, as will be seen later. By and large, the influence of the center is greater than that of the surround, so a diffuse light usually produces an attenuated form of the center response.

Experimental evidence from several species suggests that the surround of a bipolar cell's receptive field is established by horizontal cells. For example, direct injection of hyperpolarizing current into horizontal cells, which mimics the effect of light, hyperpolarizes on-center bipolar cells and depolarizes off-center bipolar cells. The latency of the bipolar cell's response to surround illumination corresponds to the latency of the horizontal cell's response. The size of the surround is correlated with the total size of the horizontal cells' receptive fields, which are very large, because horizontal cells tend to be electrically coupled to one another. Drugs that decrease the electrical coupling between horizontal cells also decrease the size of the bipolar cell's receptive-field surround. The synaptic connections mediating these interactions between horizontal cells and bipolar cells are incompletely understood. The horizontal cells could act directly on the bipolar cell's dendrites or indirectly by way of the photoreceptors themselves.

The synaptic terminals of bipolar cells make characteristic contacts, called dyad junctions, in the inner plexiform layer (Figure 6.5). Opposite a synaptic ribbon in the bipolar cell's terminal (large solid arrow) there are always two postsynaptic profiles. One of these is usually an amacrine cell, and the other may be an amacrine cell or a ganglion cell. The postsynaptic amacrine profile may also be presynaptic to its bipolar-cell input, an arrangement called a reciprocal synapse (open arrow in Figure 6.5). Such a feedback circuit would be ideally situated to modulate the membrane potential of the bipolar cell's terminal as a function of that cell's effect on the amacrine cell. If the bipolar cell excited the amacrine cell, which in turn inhibited the bipolar cell, the feedback would be negative.

Properties of Amacrine Cells and Interplexiform Cells

Amacrine cells, so named because they generally lack identifiable axons, participate in what are perhaps the most complex circuits in the retina. They exhibit a bewildering array of morphological types (e.g., more than 20 in the cat), and they have been shown to contain a variety of substances that can serve as synaptic messengers. Intracellular recordings from amacrine cells indicate that some, though not all, generate action potentials. The responses may be either transient or sustained in character. Amacrine cells exhibit on-, off-, and on–off-type receptive fields, which in some cases correspond in size, more or less, to the spread of the cells' processes in the inner plexiform layer. The connections of amacrine cells indicate that they are responsible for lateral interactions in the inner plexiform layer, but few functions can be definitely assigned to them. One role of the AII amacrine cell is known and will be discussed later.

Interplexiform cells differ from amacrine cells in that, in addition to their contacts with amacrine and bipolar cells, they send processes into the outer plexiform layer, where they contact horizontal cells. They thus appear to mediate interactions between the two major classes of interneurons in the two plexiform layers. In the goldfish, this cell class contains dopamine and is presynaptic and postsynaptic to amacrine cells in the inner nuclear layer, and presynaptic principally to horizontal cells in the outer nuclear layer. It is possible that dopamine released from these cells modulates the sizes of bipolar cells' receptive fields by reducing the electrical coupling between horizontal cells.

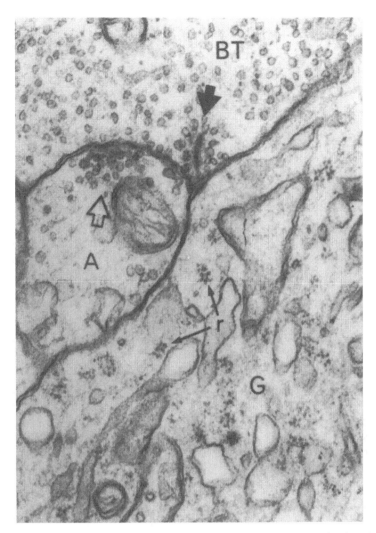

Figure 6.5. Electron micrograph of a dyad junction in the inner plexiform layer of the human retina. BT, bipolar-cell terminal; A, amacrine cell; G, ganglion cell; r, ribosome particles; large black arrow, synaptic ribbon; large open arrow, reciprocal synapse from amacrine cell to bipolar-cell terminal. (Reprinted from J. E. Dowling: Organization of vertebrate retinas. *Investigative Ophthalmology and Visual Science* 9:655–680, 1970, with permission of the Association for Research in Vision and Ophthalmology.)

Receptive Fields of Ganglion Cells

Depolarization in bipolar cells results, as a rule, in depolarization of the ganglion cells with which they establish synaptic contact. Thus, the synapse between a bipolar cell and a ganglion cell is sign-conserving or excitatory in both the on and off channels. These synapses are located in the inner plexiform layer, which is divided into two major sublaminae. The terminals of off bipolar cells ramify nearest the inner nuclear layer in sublamina *a* (the off sublamina), whereas the on bipolar cells distribute their terminals nearer the ganglion cell layer in sublamina *b* (the on sublamina) (Figure 6.6). The centers of the receptive fields of ganglion cells correspond approximately in size to the spread of their dendrites in the inner plexiform layer, but this correlation is not exact. Amacrine cell inputs undoubtedly contribute to the receptive fields of ganglion cells in various ways, but few of these are understood in any detail.

Two common types of ganglion cells restrict their dendritic arbors to either the on sublamina or off sublamina of the inner plexiform layer and exhibit the receptive-field characteristics of their bipolar-cell inputs. Thus, some ganglion cells have on-center, off-surround receptive fields, and others have off-center, on-surround receptive fields (Figure 6.7A). As is the case for bipolar cells, the center and surround of the receptive field are mutually antagonistic. Diffuse light usually evokes an attenuated version of the response to a central spot. Ganglion cells are often referred to simply in terms of their center responses; thus, one speaks of on-center or off-center ganglion cells.

There is now evidence that the center–surround organization illustrated in Figure 6.7A is the result of complex input circuitry that can be schematized as in Figure 6.7B. A strong "center mechanism" dominates the central region of the receptive field and presumably represents the direct synaptic contacts between bipolar cells and the ganglion cell's dendrites. A relatively weaker "surround mechanism" extends through and beyond the central part of the receptive field. Even though the surround mechanism coexists with that of the center, the latter is much stronger and dictates the responses to centered stimuli. The surround mechanism probably comprises contributions from the bipolar cells' surrounds, as well as influences from amacrine cells. The algebraic sum of the center and surround mechanisms (Figure 6.7B, lower panel) has a vague resemblance to a sombrero with a tall peak, so this model of the receptive field is sometimes called the "Mexican-hat model." When the spatial profiles of center and surround mechanisms can be described by Gaussian functions, as is sometimes the case, the model is referred to as the "difference-of-Gaussians model."

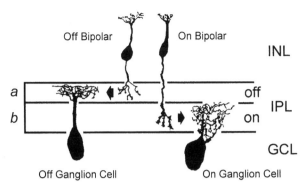

Figure 6.6. On and off sublaminae of the inner plexiform layer. Off-center (flat) bipolar cells distribute their dendrites in sublamina *a* of the inner plexiform layer, and on-center (invaginating) bipolars distribute their dendrites in sublamina *b*. Ganglion cells with dendrites restricted to one or the other of these sublaminae inherit the basic receptive-field pattern of the bipolar cells providing their input. (Adapted from E. V. Famiglietti, Jr., and H. Kolb: Structural basis for on- and off-responses in retinal ganglion cells. *Science* 194:193–5. Copyright 1976, with permission of the American Association for the Advancement of Science.)

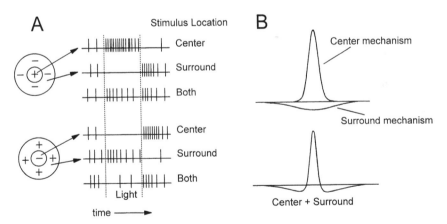

Figure 6.7. (A) Two types of ganglion cell receptive fields. Top: on-center, off-surround field. Bottom: off-center, on-surround field. Traces in each panel illustrate the effects on the action-potential frequency of stimulating the center, the surround, and both simultaneously. Plus signs, on responses; minus signs, off responses. (B) Mexican-hat model or difference-of-Gaussians model of the center–surround receptive field. This model derives from evidence that the surround mechanism extends through and beyond the center of the receptive field. The strength of each mechanism's effect on the cell is indicated by the height of the curve above the baseline.

On–Off Receptive Fields with Complex Properties

Some ganglion cells have dendrites that ramify in both the on and off sublaminae of the inner plexiform layer, giving the cells access to excitatory input at both the onset and offset of a light spot anywhere in their receptive fields. Amacrine cells with processes ramifying in both the on and off sublaminae of the inner plexiform layer could also provide excitatory on–off inputs to ganglion cells.

Some ganglion cells with on–off receptive fields exhibit a preference for stimuli moving in a particular direction, a property called directional preference or, more commonly, directional selectivity. Note that the cell in Figure 6.8A responds to movements in many directions, but generates the largest response to movement in one direction, the preferred direction. The minimal response is evoked by movement in the null direction, which is usually opposite the preferred direction.

A hypothetical circuit that could account for directional selectivity is illustrated in Figure 6.8B. Two amacrine cells, one inhibitory and the other excitatory, establish the preferred and null axes. When a stimulus moves across the receptive field from right to left, the excitatory amacrine cell is activated first and causes the ganglion cell to fire. When the stimulus moves in the null direction (i.e., from left to right), the inhibitory amacrine cell vetoes any response that might arise because of input from the excitatory amacrine cell. This circuit is sensitive to the sequence of activation of the two types of amacrine cells and bestows a directional preference on the ganglion cell. Although the circuit in Figure 6.8B is conjectural, it is believed that amacrine cells are responsible for such behavior, because directionally selective responses are not observed in receptors, horizontal cells, or bipolar cells. Note also that the amacrine cells of Figure 6.8B would not be directionally selective themselves; in this case the selectivity emerges from the neural connections and is not simply a property of the presynaptic elements.

Circuitry of the Rod Pathway

In the mammalian retina, rod signals reach the ganglion cells by a less direct route than do cone signals. When APB (which blocks normal synaptic transmission between receptors and on bipolar cells) is applied to the cat's retina and stimuli are used that affect cones, only the on response is eliminated in retinal ganglion cells. In contrast, when the retina is dark-adapted and one applies stimuli that affect only rods, both on responses and off responses are eliminated by this drug. This indicates that rod bipolar cells are depolarized by light, a conclusion supported by intracel-

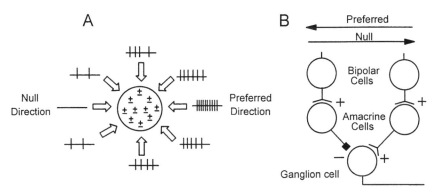

Figure 6.8. (A) Diagrammatic representation of a directionally selective ganglion cell. Open arrows indicate the movement direction of the stimulus spot across the receptive field. These cells often give on (+) and off (−) responses to stimuli flashed anywhere in their receptive fields. (B) Hypothetical circuit for directional selectivity.

lular recordings in some animals. If the rod bipolar cell is depolarized by light, how do ganglion cells acquire their off responses in the dark-adapted retina?

A combination of electrophysiologic and anatomic methods has demonstrated that rod input to the ganglion cells in mammals is mediated by the AII amacrine cell, which essentially splits the rod bipolar signal and injects it into the cone bipolar pathways (Figure 6.9). The AII amacrine cell is depolarized by the rod bipolar cell's neurotransmitter and uses the inhibitory transmitter glycine to hyperpolarize the synaptic terminal of the cone off bipolar cell, and probably the dendrite of the off-center ganglion cell as well. Through these sign-inverting synapses, the depolarization of the AII amacrine cell is converted to hyperpolarization of the cone off bipolar cell and the off-center ganglion cell. These latter two cells are then depolarized at light offset, just as they are when driven by the cone pathway. The AII amacrine cell depolarizes the synaptic terminal of the cone on bipolar cell by electrical coupling through a gap junction, and the cone on bipolar cell depolarizes the ganglion cell through its normal chemical synapse. This means that the ganglion cells are third-order neurons in the cone pathway, but at least fourth-order neurons in the rod pathway.

Disposition of Ganglion Cells and Their Receptive Fields on the Retina

Ganglion cells often are not distributed uniformly across the retina, but have their highest spatial densities in areas subserving acute vision. The

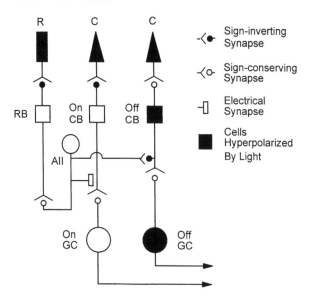

Figure 6.9. Circuitry of the mammalian rod pathway. R, rod; C, cone; RB, rod bipolar; CB, cone bipolar; AII, a specific type of amacrine cell; GC, ganglion cell.

area centralis of the cat's retina and the visual streak in the rabbit are two such regions. Ganglion cell density decreases with distance from these areas, and usually there is a reciprocal relationship between the spatial density of a particular class of ganglion cells and the average size of the cells' receptive fields. For example, the smallest receptive fields in the primate retina are located in the fovea, which is served by the largest number of ganglion cells per unit area of the retina (even though these are displaced to the side of the foveal pit). Receptive-field size increases with distance from the fovea as ganglion cell density decreases.

The retina is literally carpeted by the receptive fields of the ganglion cells, and any retinal point lies within the receptive fields of many ganglion cells. Where there are specialized types of cells, each retinal point lies in the receptive field of at least one, and often more than one, representative of each type. In particular, the receptive fields of both on-center and off-center ganglion cells overlap to such a degree that information about what is happening at any point on the retina is encoded in the discharge of both classes of cells.

The term coverage factor or simply coverage is used by anatomists to signify the number of cells of a particular class whose dendrites overlap at a given retinal point. To a physiologist, the term refers to the number of cells whose receptive-field centers overlap at a given point. Because receptive-field centers usually have dimensions comparable to the cells' dendritic fields, the two approaches often yield the same numbers for a given class of cells. In principle, there is no reason to exclude the receptive field's surround from the estimate of coverage, because the discharge of a ganglion cell can be modulated through the surround as well as the center of its receptive field. In fact, the cells that "see" a retinal point are those influenced through any part of the receptive field. The area containing such cells has been called the point image, which differs from coverage in being an area rather than a number. These concepts will be discussed in more detail in a later chapter.

On and Off Responses, Lateral Inhibition, and Contrast Enhancement

The functional significance of lateral inhibition and the carpeting of the retina by ganglion cell receptive fields can be appreciated by observing what happens at a black/white border. Consider a population of on-center ganglion cells, of which four are depicted in Figure 6.10. Two of these are near the border, and two are some distance from it. Observe that cell A fires at a higher rate than cell D because the receptive-field center dominates a cell's response to diffuse illumination. Furthermore, cell B has a higher rate of discharge than cell A, because only part of its inhibitory surround is illuminated. Conversely, cell C has a lower discharge rate than cell D, because one part of its inhibitory surround is illuminated. The net effect is to create a pattern of activity that accentuates the difference between the firing rates of the on-center cells just at the border. If an increase in the activity of these on-center cells is interpreted by the brain as "there is more light here," then one should see a very bright zone to the left of the border and a very dark zone to the right. Such zones, called Mach bands, are readily observed when viewing a sharp black/white border. If one considers the carpet of off-center cells and assumes that an increase in their discharge means "there is less light here," the same bands of contrast enhancement are predicted.

Figure 6.11 illustrates another perceptual phenomenon that possibly can be traced to the center–surround organization of retinal receptive fields. In this Hermann grid, dark spots appear at the intersections of the white strips separating the black squares. Consider the two on-center cells with receptive fields located as illustrated. The one centered in the intersection will have a lower discharge rate than the one outside the intersection, because more of its off surround is illuminated. If the discharge of this cell means "light here," the brain would interpret the different firing

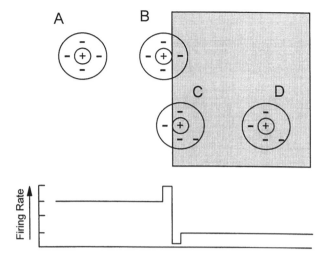

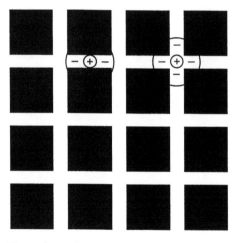

Figure 6.10. Contrast enhancement by center–surround receptive fields.

Figure 6.11. The Hermann grid. The receptive fields of two on-center ganglion cells are illustrated, one at an intersection of the white lines separating the black squares, the other between two intersections.

rates of these two cells to mean "more light between than at the intersections," which is what one sees. The off-center cells have a complementary distribution of activity, but would send an equivalent message to the brain: "darker at than between the intersections." When the Hermann grid is constructed of white squares on a black background, the illusion has the opposite contrast; there are light spots in the intersections.

The presence of lateral inhibition makes the retinal neurons especially sensitive to local variations in illuminance or, what is the same thing, to local spatial contrast. Note also that the mutual antagonism between center and surround reduces the effectiveness of diffuse illumination and prevents the cell's response from saturating at high luminance levels. This permits the cell to continue to respond to local contrast over a wide range of ambient light levels.

Neurotransmitters and Neuromodulators in the Retina

Nerve cells of the retina, like those in the brain, generally communicate with each other by chemical means. Electrical coupling does occur, as already noted for the case of the AII amacrine cell, but it appears to be used for very selected types of contact. Messenger substances active in the retina include acetylcholine, biogenic amines such as dopamine and serotonin, amino acids such as glutamate and glycine, and peptides such as substance P and somatostatin.

The rapid signaling required for high-fidelity transmission of information about changing patterns of illumination is achieved by conventional neurotransmitters, of which glutamate is a good example. This is likely to be the transmitter contained in photoreceptor terminals. The major inhibitory transmitters of the retina are glycine and γ-aminobutyric acid (GABA), with the latter occurring in large numbers of amacrine cells. Acetylcholine is also present in certain classes of amacrine cells in some animals. The neurotransmitters present in a given cell type vary considerably among species.

Slower processes affecting retinal circuitry are mediated by substances most accurately called neuromodulators. These include peptide molecules and dopamine. The roles of the neuromodulators in vision probably are diverse and at the moment are rather obscure, but it is likely that these substances are important for such functions as light and dark adaptation.

Light and Dark Adaptation: The Duplex Retina

One of the most important characteristics of the visual system is its ability to function over a wide range of ambient light levels. As one moves from nearly total darkness to bright sunlight on snow, the level of illumination increases by a factor of 10 billion. Various mechanisms contribute to the eye's large dynamic range, including the pupillary light reflex, which decreases the amount of light entering the eye by reducing pupil diameter.

Animals with slit pupils can essentially obliterate the eye's aperture. The circular pupil in humans can decrease in diameter from 8 mm to 2 mm, reducing its area by a factor of 16. Clearly, this cannot account for the capacity of the human eye to function efficiently over the full range of illumination that it encounters. To accomplish this, the eyes of humans and other animals use several mechanisms, all included in the machinery of the retina.

Animals that are active both day and night, such as humans, have two types of photoreceptors, one suited for low and the other for high light levels. Under dark-adapted conditions (scotopic vision), the highly sensitive rods permit the eye to see dim objects. When light levels are high (photopic vision), various adaptive mechanisms render the rods less sensitive than the cones, which then dominate the responses of the retina to light. Figuratively speaking, then, the human eye can switch between two retinas, one for low light levels and the other for high, and for this reason the human retina is said to be duplex. "Switching" may not be exactly the right word, because both the rod and cone systems can operate at the same time under some conditions. When the retina is dark-adapted, the rods are the most sensitive, but the cones respond to stimuli that are sufficiently bright. This is why we can see the colors of neon lights on dark nights.

Rods are absent from the primate fovea, so the most sensitive region in the dark-adapted retina lies about 18–20° from the fovea, where the rod density peaks (Figure 6.12). For this reason, it is easiest to see a very dim star in the night sky by looking slightly away from it, so that the image falls on the parafoveal zone of high rod density. In the light-adapted retina, the point of lowest threshold is the fovea, where cone density is highest.

As the eye adapts to light, the part of the spectrum to which the eye is most sensitive shifts toward longer wavelengths. This phenomenon, called the Purkinje shift, is due to the fact that some cones are responsive to longer wavelengths than rods. Because the rods contain only one photopigment, rhodopsin, they cannot distinguish between different wavelengths of light. Thus, color vision is mediated exclusively by cones, so lights that are too dim to stimulate cones are not seen as colored.

The fovea of the human eye has a number of specializations that give it the highest spatial resolution of any part of the retina (see Chapter 9). One of these is that the foveal cones are densely packed (Figure 6.12) and very thin. Moreover, foveal cones are linked to midget bipolar cells and midget ganglion cells, which, in the central part of the retina, provide an exclusive channel to the brain for a single photoreceptor. Rods, on the other hand, are most numerous outside the fovea, and the activities of

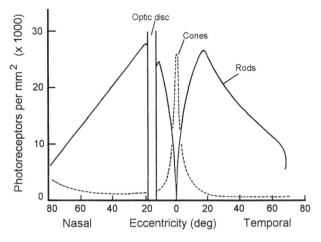

Figure 6.12. Distribution of rods and cones along a horizontal line through the fovea. (Adapted from J. L. Brown, after Woodson: The structure of the visual system. In *Vision and Visual Perception*, ed. C. H. Graham, pp. 39–59. New York: Wiley-Liss. Copyright 1954, with permission of Wiley-Liss, Inc., a subsidiary of John Wiley & Sons.)

many rods are combined in the inputs to bipolar and ganglion cells. Consequently, the retina has its highest spatial resolution at the fovea if the incident light levels are capable of influencing cones. In the dark-adapted state, spatial resolution declines for stimuli so dim as to affect only rods.

If the human eye has been exposed to light for a while and the light is then extinguished, the threshold for detecting a flash declines along the so-called dark adaptation curve (Figure 6.13). For a while, the cones are the most sensitive elements, and their adaptation can be followed if stimuli are restricted to the fovea. At some point the rods become more sensitive than the cones, and the threshold descends along another limb of the curve that can be seen in isolation in individuals whose retinas contain no cones (rod monochromats). At the inflection point, where the two curves intersect, photopic vision gives way to scotopic vision. The major characteristics of these two states are summarized in Table 6.1.

Network and Receptor Adaptation

Additional mechanisms operate within both photopic vision and scotopic vision to modulate the eye's sensitivity, each contributing to the adaptation observed at a given light level. These can be separated into processes occurring in the synaptic networks of the retina (network adaptation) and those taking place in the photoreceptors themselves (receptor adaptation).

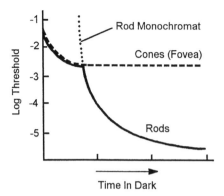

Figure 6.13. Time course of dark adaptation. The cone curve can be measured by restricting stimulation to the fovea. A rod monochromat generates only the rod portion of the curve.

Table 6.1. *Comparison of scotopic vision and photopic vision*

Rod or scotopic vison	Cone or photopic vision
High sensitivity	Low sensitivity
Parafoveal sensitivity highest	Foveal sensitivity highest
Poor acuity	Good acuity
No color vision	Color vision
More sensitive to short wavelengths	More sensitive to long wavelengths

The distinction between these two processes may be thought of in terms of the scheme in Figure 6.14. Mechanisms in each compartment set a gain or amplification factor that determines the size of the output for a given input. This factor is, in turn, controlled by feedback reflecting the activity in each compartment. In the photoreceptor, the gain is reduced as background light levels increase and more photopigment is bleached. The gain of the network compartment is decreased as signal traffic through its circuitry increases. A major goal of retinal research is to understand the cellular and synaptic mechanisms responsible for the variable gains of the two compartments.

Study of the cellular processes underlying adaptation has been greatly aided by the technique of reflection or retinal densitometry (Figure 6.15). When a beam of light is projected into the living eye, some of it is reflected back and exits through the pupil, after having passed twice

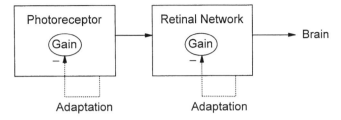

Figure 6.14. Schematic representation of the process of receptor adaptation and network adaptation. The two processes are shown as two compartments with separate negative-feedback mechanisms to decrease their gain or amplification as light intensity increases.

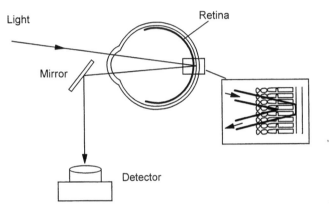

Figure 6.15. Method of reflection densitometry.

through the photoreceptors. With suitable equipment, this reflected light can be used to measure the density and spectral characteristics of the photopigments. The method allows simultaneous assessment of visual thresholds and bleaching of visual pigments in the living human eye. At very low light levels, thresholds increase before there is any detectable bleaching of photopigment. Clearly, some pigment molecules are being bleached, but their numbers are below the limits of detection. Because a decrease in photopigment concentration is not limiting the sensitivity of the retina at these low light levels, the changes in threshold must be due to adjustments within the neural circuits; hence the term "network adaptation." The existence of network adaptation is also supported by experiments in the skate (a marine ray) showing that the electrical responses of proximal retinal neurons (bipolar cells and ganglion cells) are affected by dim adapting lights that have no detectable influence on photoreceptor sensitivity.

As background light levels increase, several adaptational processes operate within the photoreceptor cells to set the overall responsiveness of the retina. The great sensitivity of the rod limits its operating range to fairly low levels of ambient light. At high light levels, the number of open cation channels in the rod decreases to the point that no further decrease can occur, so quantal absorptions no longer produce a detectable hyperpolarizing response to incremental stimulation. This phenomenon, called rod saturation, cannot account fully for the light-induced decrease in rod sensitivity, because significant adaptation develops at light levels below those required for saturation. Other mechanisms are at work to reduce the sensitivity of both rods and cones.

The absorption of a quantum of light by a photoreceptor not only initiates the enzymatic cascade that results in the closing of the cation channels but also triggers a number of processes to reverse the effects of this absorption (see Chapter 4). If other photons arrive at short intervals, they act on a system that has been changed by the previous absorption events. For instance, intracellular calcium concentrations are lower than in the dark-adapted state because of the decreased influx but continued extrusion of this cation. Calcium influences the activities of a variety of proteins that determine the rates at which critical enzymatic processes occur. Although these processes are not yet fully understood, the resulting changes reduce the hyperpolarizing effect of subsequent quantal absorptions, in effect reducing the gain of the photoreceptor. The same or different processes displace the receptor's membrane potential toward depolarized levels, permitting additional hyperpolarizing responses to be registered.

Reflection densitometry has identified one factor that appears to play an important role in receptor adaptation. When a moderately intense adapting light is extinguished, the threshold drops instantly, presumably because of the rapid disappearance of network adaptation, and reaches a "floor" level from which it decreases slowly. During the slower phase of dark adaptation, the logarithm of the threshold decreases with the same time course as the percentage of bleached photopigment. Studies in a variety of animals have shown that if the retina is separated from the pigment epithelium, photopigment cannot regenerate, and the receptor phase of dark adaptation does not occur.

It is not yet known how the presence of bleached pigment reduces the responsiveness of the photoreceptor. It cannot be simply that the concentration of unbleached pigment is inadequate to absorb the impinging quanta. Bleaching 50% of the rhodopsin should lower the sensitivity by a factor of 2 on the basis of a simple reduction in quantum catch, but this much bleaching actually reduces sensitivity by a factor of 100 or more in the skate retina.

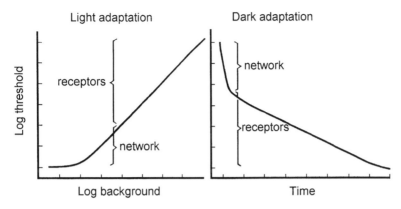

Figure 6.16. Schematic summary of the contributions of network and receptor mechanisms to light and dark adaptations in the skate retina. (Reprinted from J. E. Dowling: Receptoral and network mechanisms in visual adaptation. *Neuroscience Research Program Bulletin* 15:397–406, 1977, with permission of MIT Press. Copyright 1977 by the Massachusetts Institute of Technology.)

Figure 6.16, based on studies in the skate retina by John Dowling, provides a useful summary of the contributions of network and receptor mechanisms to retinal sensitivity during light and dark adaptation. When the retina is exposed to low levels of adapting light, network mechanisms account for the greater part of the adjustment of sensitivity (Figure 6.16, left). As light levels increase, receptor adaptation assumes an increasingly greater role in the process. When the light is turned off, network adaptation disappears quickly, followed by a long period of slower adaptation, during which the threshold decreases as the fraction of bleached pigment decreases (Figure 6.16, right).

Retinomotor Movements

In invertebrates and many cold-blooded vertebrates, the eye can also adapt to different levels of illumination by movement of screening pigments and by changes in length of the photoreceptors themselves. Such retinomotor movements have been extensively studied in teleost fish. In the dark, contractile elements in the rods shorten, pulling the outer segments away from the shielding effect of melanin granules in the pigment epithelium. At the same time, the cones lengthen, and their outer segments retreat into the pigment epithelium. These processes reverse in the light. Pigment granules also migrate within the pigment epithelium, occupying exten-

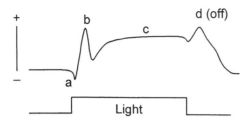

Figure 6.17. Schematic representation of the ERG.

sions around the outer segments in light, and moving back toward the sclera in the dark.

The Electroretinogram

Many studies of retinal function, such as its behavior during light and dark adaptation, have exploited the fact that electrodes positioned so as to record the voltage difference between the cornea and some reference point register a complex waveform in response to a light stimulus (Figure 6.17). The various components of this electroretinogram (ERG) have been traced, in part at least, to the responses of particular retinal elements.

The earliest deviation, the a-wave, persists following occlusion of the central retinal artery (and retinal circulation) and behaves in other ways as though it were generated by the photoreceptors themselves. Only the beginning of the photoreceptors' response is revealed in the a-wave, because later phases are obscured by the activities of more proximal elements.

The b-wave is eliminated by occlusion of the central retinal artery and is therefore generated by elements central to the photoreceptors. Experimental evidence suggests that it reflects bipolar-cell activity but is primarily due to glial cells (Müller cells). These cells sequester K^+ from the extracellular space, so their membrane currents reflect the activity of the neurons surrounding them. Activity of the bipolar cells changes the K^+ concentration in the extracellular space, and this modifies the membrane potential of the Müller cells, giving rise to the b-wave.

Intracellular recordings from the pigment epithelium indicate that these cells give rise to the c-wave. In the dark-adapted retina, the spectral sensitivity of the c-wave is that of rhodopsin, not melanin, indicating that the pigment epithelium is responding to some process originating with the photoreceptors. The c-wave is thought to arise from the pigment epithelium as a result of changes in extracellular K^+ due to illumination of the photoreceptors, in a fashion similar to the way the activity of cells in the inner retina influences the membrane potential of the Müller cells to produce the b-wave. There is little or no d-wave or off component in the rod-dominated eye of the cat, whereas this wave is prominent in the cone-dominated eyes of the ground squirrel. This suggests that the d-wave reflects, in part at least, the depolarization of off bipolar cells, which would be sparse in the cat but common in the ground squirrel.

Further Reading

Barlow, H. B., and Levick, W. R. (1965). The mechanism of directionally selective units in rabbit's retina. *Journal of Physiology* 178:477–504.

Brecha, N., Eldred, W., Kuljis, R. O., and Karten, H. J. (1984). Identification and localization of biologically active peptides in the vertebrate retina. In *Progress in Retinal Research*, vol. 3, ed. N. N. Osborne and B. Chade, pp. 185–226. Oxford: Pergamon Press.

Burkhardt, D. (1993). Synaptic feedback, depolarization, and color opponency in cone photoreceptors. *Visual Neuroscience* 10:981–9.

Dowling, J. E. (1987). *The Retina*. Cambridge: Harvard University Press.

Fain, G. L., and Matthews, H. R. (1990). Calcium and the mechanism of light adaptation in vertebrate photoreceptors. *Trends in Neurosciences* 13:378–84.

Rodieck, R. W. (1973). *The Vertebrate Retina*. San Francisco: Freeman.

Schiller, P. H. (1992). The ON and OFF channels of the visual system. *Trends in Neurosciences* 15:86–92.

Wässle, H., and Boycott, B. B. (1991). Functional architecture of the mammalian retina. *Physiological Reviews* 71:447–80.

CHAPTER 7

THE RETINO-GENICULATE PROJECTION

All information about the retinal image that is directly available to the brain is transmitted by the axons of retinal ganglion cells. In higher mammals, and particularly primates, the projection to the cortex via the lateral geniculate nucleus of the thalamus appears to be essential for conscious visual perception. Retinal axons also reach the hypothalamus, superior colliculus, pretectum, and various other nuclei of the brain stem and diencephalon that subserve a variety of functions, such as reflex orientation to visual stimuli, stabilization of gaze, and control of pupil diameter. This chapter focuses primarily on the retino-geniculate component of the projection to the cerebral cortex, but several of the principles dealt with here are relevant to brain-stem projections as well.

Parallel Processing of the Retinal Image and Classes of Ganglion Cells

Previous chapters have shown how the retinal circuitry establishes one channel to signal increments and another to signal decrements of illumination. These on and off channels encode complementary versions of the distribution of light on the retina and transmit them in parallel to the central nervous system. Also, as discussed earlier, other features of the retinal image, such as movement direction, can be signaled by specialized ganglion cells. Thus, the retinal image is not transmitted in raw form to the brain, but is analyzed in different ways by different ganglion cells, which then communicate their "views" of the image along separate channels. Different animals segregate different aspects of the retinal image as part of this strategy of parallel processing. The visual systems of the macaque monkey and the cat have been studied most thoroughly in this respect, and they will be described here in some detail to illustrate both the similarities and differences between two mammalian species.

A major clue that a retina contains different functional classes of ganglion cells is the observation that the conduction velocities and diameters of axons in the optic tract fall into distinct groups. Similar clusterings in cutaneous and muscle nerves have long been known to reflect the presence of axons with different functions. In addition to axonal properties, various other features serve to identify different functional classes of retinal ganglion cells, including perikaryal and dendritic morphology, receptive-field properties, and central projections.

Our knowledge of retinal cells has developed from two parallel methodological approaches – the morphologic and physiologic. Thus, anatomists have developed classification schemes based on the structural characteristics of cells, while physiologists have grouped cells into categories with similar response properties. Often the result has been that two (or more) systems of nomenclature have emerged to describe the retinal cells in a given species. Fortunately, it is often possible to show that a given morphologic class corresponds to a particular physiologic class of cells, but in some cases the correlations are not perfect, and all classification schemes evolve as new information is acquired.

Retinal Ganglion Cells and Their Central Projections in Primates

Approximately 90% of retinal ganglion cells in the macaque monkey, whose vision is very similar to that of humans, belong to one of two classes that possess receptive fields with antagonistic center–surround organization (Table 7.1). P cells (about 80% of the population) take their name from the fact that their axons terminate in the parvocellular layers of the LGN, whereas the axons of retinal M cells (10% of the population) terminate in the magnocellular layers. (The layers of the LGN are discussed later.) Perhaps the most striking difference between M and P cells is that in certain species the latter are connected to cones in such a way as to be excited by some wavelengths of light and inhibited by others. Such P cells are sometimes described as color-opponent; M cells, which are indifferent to the wavelength of the illumination, are characterized as broadband. Other properties that distinguish between these two cell types are listed in Table 7.1. It should be noted that the retinas of nocturnal primate species, such as the bush baby, are dominated by rods and contain P cells

Table 7.1. *Classes and properties of retinal ganglion cells in the macaque monkey*

Property	M cell (10%)	P cell (80%)	Other (10%)
Morphology	parasol	midget or bistratified	variable
Soma size	large	intermediate	small
Receptive field	center/surround	center/surround	variable
Color opponency	no	yes	no
Axon conduction velocity	fast	intermediate	slow
LGN target	magnocellular	parvocellular	koniocellular
Other targets	SC, PT[a]	none	SC, LGN

[a]SC, superior colliculus; PT, pretectum.

that are not color-opponent. The central projections of retinal M and P cells to their direct targets in the brain stem and thalamus, and beyond to the cerebral cortex, are conventionally referred to as the M and P pathways, respectively.

By and large, M and P cells appear to correspond respectively to the parasol and midget ganglion cells originally described by Ramón y Cajal. Figure 7.1 illustrates two such cells from a human retina. However, this correlation is not perfect; for instance, the ganglion cell carrying chromatic signals from the short-wavelength cones is not a midget cell, but nonetheless projects to the parvocellular layers. To avoid confusion, we shall use the M- and P-cell designations based on the pattern of termination in the LGN, but it should be kept in mind that the terminology applied to these pathways is provisional, and new information may require changes.

The remaining 10% of macaque retinal ganglion cells form a heterogeneous, small-bodied group that is poorly understood. Many of these cells project to the superior colliculus, but others send their axons to the LGN, where they contact cells lying outside the parvocellular and magnocellular laminae. As discussed later, these cells may constitute a third, small cell pathway from the primate retina.

The parvocellular and magnocellular laminae stand out prominently in a coronal section through the macaque LGN stained for cell bodies. In the part of the nucleus representing the binocular visual field there are six such layers, four parvocellular and two magnocellular. Magnocellular layers 1 and 2 are ventral and nearest the optic tract, and parvocellular layers 3–6 lie dorsally. "Magno" and "parvo" refer to the relative sizes of the perikarya of the neurons in the different layers. The contralateral eye projects

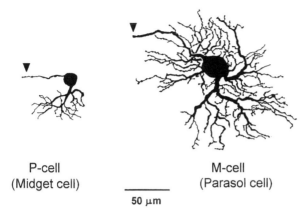

P-cell
(Midget cell)

M-cell
(Parasol cell)

_____
50 μm

Figure 7.1. Examples of midget and parasol ganglion cells from the periphery of the human retina. These presumably represent the anatomic correlates of human M and P cells, respectively. Golgi-impregnated flat mounts. Arrowheads indicate axons. (Adapted from R. W. Rodieck, K. F. Binmoeller, and J. Dineen: Parasol and midget ganglion cells of the human retina. *Journal of Comparative Neurology* 233:115–32, 1985, with permission of Wiley-Liss, Inc., a subsidiary of John Wiley & Sons.)

to layers 1, 4, and 6, and the ipsilateral eye projects to layers 2, 3, and 5 (Figure 7.2). As noted earlier, the axons of retinal P cells terminate in the parvocellular layers, and those of retinal M cells terminate in the magnocellular layers. The geniculate neurons preserve the basic properties of their retinal inputs. Thus, cells of the parvocellular layers may exhibit color-opponent properties, whereas those of the magnocellular layers are broadband in their responses.

Not so evident in the usual Nissl-stained sections are very small cells intercalated between the main laminae and also located ventrally in what are called the superficial laminae. Similar cells are found in other primate species, although the patterns of their physical distributions differ. When stained for enzymes that label them exclusively, these small cells are found to make up about 10% of the geniculate relay neurons and likely participate in a third, koniocellular, retino-cortical pathway in the primate, so named because of the tiny size of the cells.

Retinal Ganglion Cells and Their Central Projections in the Cat

Axons in the cat's optic tract form three groups based on their diameters and conduction velocities. W cells have the smallest axons and slowest conduction velocities, and Y cells have the largest axons and fastest conduction velocities. The axonal properties of X cells are intermediate be-

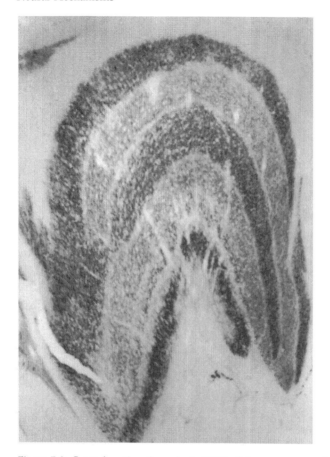

Figure 7.2. Coronal section through the LGN of the macaque monkey stained for the mitochondrial enzyme cytochrome oxidase. The darkly stained cell bodies of magnocellular layer 1 are located inferiorly. Tetrodotoxin injected into the ipsilateral eye blocked all retinal input to layers 2, 3, and 5, resulting in less enzymatic activity and lighter staining. (Courtesy of Dr. Stewart Hendry.)

tween those of W cells and Y cells. Extensive studies have added a substantial list of other features that distinguish these physiologic groups from one another (Table 7.2). X and Y cells correspond respectively to the anatomists' beta and alpha classes of retinal ganglion cells (Figure 7.3). Whereas the X and Y groups are relatively homogeneous, the W category comprises a number of physiologic and morphologic subgroups that probably constitute distinct functional classes. This heterogeneity is evident in

Table 7.2. *Classes and properties of retinal ganglion cells in the cat*

Property	Y cell (10%)	X cell (40%)	W cell (50%)
Morphology	alpha	beta	various
Receptive-field type	center/surround	center/surround	center/surround, on−off, other
Receptive-field size	large	small	intermediate
Axon conduction velocity	fast	intermediate	slow
Axon size	large	intermediate	small
Response to standing contrast	phasic (transient)	tonic (sustained)	variable
Edge null position	no	yes	variable
Motion sensitivity	fast	intermediate	slow
LGN targets	A, A1, C, MIN[a]	A, A1	C, MIN
Other targets	SC, PT, other[b]		SC, PT, other

[a] A, A1, C, MIN: See Figures 7.5 and 7.6 for LGN laminae.
[b] SC, superior colliculus; PT, pretectum.

the two W cells illustrated in Figure 7.3. Another classification scheme based on response properties identifies sluggish, brisk-sustained, and brisk-transient ganglion cells. For all practical purposes, these groups correspond to the W, X, and Y categories, respectively.

One of the first distinctions noted between X and Y cells is that they respond differently to a stationary grating pattern whose luminance varies sinusoidally across the receptive field. The cells can be activated by alternate presentations of the grating and a gray background or by counterphasing the grating (i.e., rapidly interchanging the dark and light stripes). X cells cease to respond to the stimulus when the grating occupies a particular position relative to the receptive field, the so-called null position (Figure 7.4 and Table 7.2). Y cells do not have such null positions, and they also respond twice during each stimulus presentation or contrast cycle, whereas X cells respond only once (Figure 7.4). These characteristic responses to grating stimuli are often used to identify the cell types during physiologic recording.

Retinofugal projections in the cat terminate in the thalamus, hypothalamus, pretectum, and midbrain. The principal thalamic terminus, the lateral geniculate complex, consists of dorsal (LGNd) and ventral (LGNv) divisions. Here we shall use LGN to designate the dorsal component only, which comprises layers A, A1, several C laminae, a medial segment called the medial interlaminar nucleus (MIN), and a rostral extension termed the

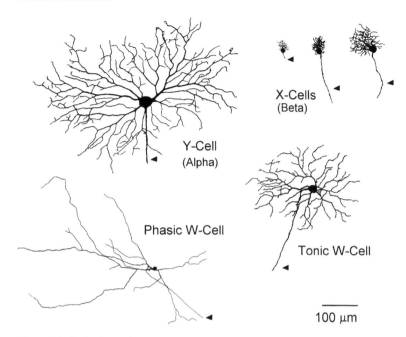

Figure 7.3. Retinal ganglion cells in the cat stained during intracellular recording and classified according to their physiologic responses. Physiologic Y cells correspond to morphologic alpha cells of the retina. The X cells, morphologic beta cells, were collected at three retinal locations of increasing distance from the area centralis, the smallest cell being located most centrally. The heterogeneous class of W cells is associated with an equally heterogeneous group of morphologic types designated gamma, delta, epsilon, and so forth. Arrowheads indicate axons. (Courtesy of Dr. L. R. Stanford. The two W cells are illustrated in L. R. Stanford: W-cells in the cat retina: correlated morphological and physiological evidence for two distinct classes. *Journal of Neurophysiology* 57:218–44, 1987. Reproduced with permission of the American Physiological Society.)

"geniculate wing" (Figure 7.5). Lamina A receives axons from the contralateral eye, and lamina A1 from the ipsilateral eye. This alternating pattern of ocular input is also present in the C laminae and in the MIN. One region of the MIN receives crossed afferents representing the ipsilateral visual field.

W, X, and Y cells do not project indiscriminately to midbrain and thalamic targets. The most important differences are noted in Table 7.2 and Figure 7.6. W cells project to the superior colliculus and pretectum and to the C laminae and the MIN of the LGN. Y cells project to the superior colliculus and pretectum and to layers A and A1, one of the C laminae, and the MIN of the LGN. X cells project principally to layers A

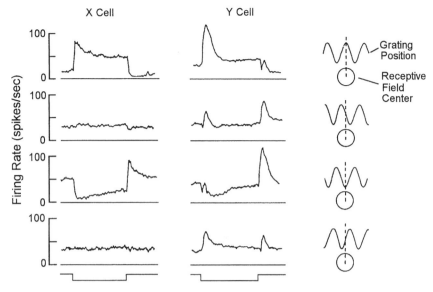

Figure 7.4. Responses of X and Y retinal ganglion cells to presentation of a sinusoidal luminance grating. Right: Relative positions of the grating and the receptive field. Left: Responses to grating turned off and on (off is down in bottom trace). Note that the X cell ceases to respond to the stimulus when the zero-crossing of the grating is near the center of the receptive field. Depending on grating position, it increases its discharge at either the onset or offset of the stimulus. The Y cell has no null position, and its discharge accelerates twice with each presentation. Traces are 2 seconds long. (Adapted from C. Enroth-Cugell and J. G. Robson: The contrast sensitivity of retinal ganglion cells of the cat. *Journal of Physiology* 187:517–52, 1966, with permission of The Physiological Society.)

and A1 of the LGN. There is little effective convergence of the different afferent types in the LGN, so the postsynaptic neurons preserve the receptive-field properties of the three types of ganglion cells. Thus, one can speak of W-, X-, and Y-type geniculate neurons in the cat.

Are There Parallels between Receptive-Field Types in Cat and Monkey?

An obvious question is whether or not certain classes of visual cells occur in all vertebrates or all mammals and subserve analogous functions. Similarities have been noted between cat Y cells and monkey M cells, and between cat X cells and monkey P cells, and cells resembling these classes have also been discerned in rabbits, rats, and other animals. Moreover, as noted earlier, recent evidence indicates that primates, like other mammals,

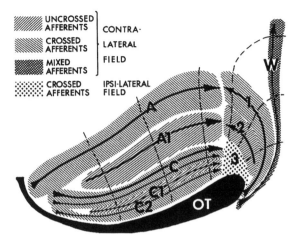

Figure 7.5. Diagrammatic illustration of a coronal section of the cat's LGN. The main laminae are designated A, A1, and the C group (C, C1, and C2). A fourth lamina, C3, does not appear to receive a direct retinal projection. Divisions of the MIN are indicated as 1, 2, and 3. W, the geniculate wing; OT, optic tract. (Reprinted from R. W. Guillery, E. E. Geisert, Jr., E. H. Polley, and C. A. Mason: An analysis of the retinal afferents to the cat's medial interlaminar nucleus and its rostral thalamic extension, the "geniculate wing." *Journal of Comparative Neurology* 194:117–42, 1980, with permission of Wiley-Liss, Inc., a subsidiary of John Wiley & Sons.)

may possess three pathways leading from the retina to the cortex. These parallels are of interest because they suggest evolutionary homology, the descent of the related classes from a common ancestor. However, the search for a commonality of function among presumably homologous cell classes has encountered difficulties. It has been pointed out, for instance, that whereas the receptive-field properties of two ganglion cell types may exhibit similarities, their patterns of central termination may differ significantly, suggesting that their roles in vision may also differ. Thus, the terminals of X and Y cells in the cat intermingle considerably in layers A and A1 of the LGN, but M and P cells of the monkey send their axons to separate laminae. There is even a tendency for on-center P cells to terminate in layers 5 and 6 and for off-center P cells to terminate in layers 3 and 4.

There are also major differences in the distributions of ganglion cell axons to different targets. W cells constitute fully half the ganglion cells of the cat's retina and provide the majority of axons terminating in the superior colliculus, whereas only about 10% of the monkey's retinal ganglion cells project to the superior colliculus. P cells of the macaque monkey

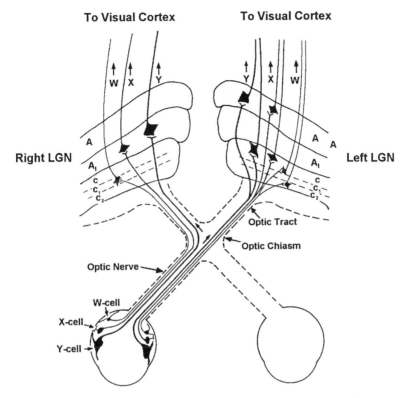

Figure 7.6. Projections from retinae to the LGN in the cat. This diagram does not show the W- and Y-cell projections to the MIN. (Reprinted from P. D. Wilson, M. H. Rowe, and J. Stone: Properties of relay cells in cat's lateral geniculate nucleus: a comparison of W-cells with X- and Y-cells. *Journal of Neurophysiology* 39:1193–209, 1976, with permission of the American Physiological Society.)

exhibit differential sensitivity to wavelength, whereas X cells in the cat do not. Most of the cat's Y cells project to the superior colliculus, but relatively few of the monkey's M cells do. These are but a few examples of the many discrepancies that urge caution in ascribing functional homology to ganglion cell classes in different species that may, indeed, derive from a common ancestor.

Research on the different classes of visual cells can be characterized as addressing two distinct questions: What aspects of their morphology and connections account for the cells' behaviors? What roles do the cells play in vision? The first question is far more tractable than the second. For instance, it is now reasonably clear how the on responses and off responses arise, but it is not certain how the brain uses these responses to appreciate increments and decrements of illumination. Similarly, the linkages between cones and cells of the parvocellular pathway in monkeys must account for the latter's differential sensitivity to light of different wavelengths, but it is not clear how the activity of these cells leads to color vision. It is likely, too, that some cells participate in more than one visual function. For instance, a single Y cell of the cat's retina may contribute synapses to two different parts of the LGN, as well as to the superior colliculus. As these structures probably serve different functions, it cannot be said that the Y cell has but one role in vision. Also, the different channels converge in a variety of patterns at various stations of the visual pathway, indicating that the brain both segregates and combines the encoded information about the retinal image in complex ways.

Retinotopic Maps in the LGN

Retinal axons terminate in an orderly fashion within the geniculate laminae, so that neighboring retinal points are represented at neighboring points in the LGN. The laminae are stacked such that cells lying along a line drawn normal to the surfaces of all the layers have their receptive fields in the same part of visual space (Figure 7.7). These cells are said to form a "projection column." In cat and monkey, the bulk of the LGN is devoted to the contralateral visual field; but in the cat, part of the MIN receives fibers from the contralateral temporal retina and therefore contains a partial map of the ipsilateral visual field (Figure 7.5). As discussed previously, the central part of the visual field has a larger representation than the peripheral field in the retinotopic geniculate map.

Effects of Stimulating the Nondominant Eye

Because of the segregation of ocular inputs in the LGN, geniculate neurons receive their principal excitatory input from only one eye, the so-called dominant eye. However, careful testing has revealed that these neurons can be influenced by signals arising from the other eye. The receptive field in the nondominant eye, which is located at a retinal site corresponding to the receptive field of the dominant eye, may contain weak excitatory and inhibitory areas. Removal of the visual cortex eliminates some but not all of the effects of stimulation of the nondominant eye, so the cortico-geniculate projection, described later, cannot account entirely for the binocular interactions observed in the LGN.

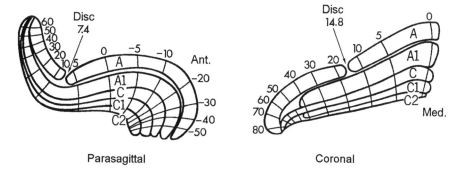

Parasagittal   Coronal

Figure 7.7. Retinotopy of the cat's LGN. The solid lines crossing the laminae indicate the positions of isoelevation (left) or isoazimuth (right) contours of the retinotopic map. Note that the regions near the horizontal and vertical meridians (0°) are relatively magnified. The map is discontinuous in layer A (nasal retina) at the position corresponding to the optic disc. (Reprinted from J. H. Kaas, R. W. Guillery, and J. M. Allman: Some principles of organization in the dorsal lateral geniculate nucleus. *Brain, Behavior and Evolution* 6:253–99, 1972, with permission of Plenum Publishing Corporation.)

Functions of LGN Lamination

Students of the visual system have long speculated about the possible functions of the lamination of the LGN, which is such a striking feature of the mammalian thalamus. W. E. Le Gros Clark suggested that the laminae segregate the primary colors of trichromatic vision, and Gordon Walls proposed that the parvocellular laminae mediate scotopic vision, and the magnocellular laminae photopic vision. Neither of these suggestions has stood the test of time. Because the laminae often segregate the terminals of different classes of retinal ganglion cells, it is clear that they lie in specialized information channels, but the patterns of segregation are not the same in different species. For instance, on channels and off channels are confined to different laminae in the ferret, but not in the cat. Also, the numbers of laminae differ between carnivores and primates.

The one consistent determinant of lamination is the ocular origin of the retinal afferents. This is all the more striking when one considers that inputs from the two eyes mix freely in other retinal targets, such as the superior colliculus and ventral LGN and are eventually joined in the binocular neurons of the visual cortex. It is difficult to avoid the conclusion that the inputs from the two eyes are kept relatively separate in the LGN as part of some process essential to binocular vision. The identity and nature of this process remain unknown.

Neural Circuitry of the LGN

As noted earlier, LGN relay cells tend to receive inputs from one or only a few retinal afferents, and consequently their receptive fields resemble those of retinal ganglion cells. In the cat, LGN relay cells are found to have W-, X-, or Y-type receptive fields, and there is preservation of the size relationships among the cell types. Thus, Y-type LGN neurons have large somata and thick axons that conduct rapidly, W-type neurons have small somata, and so forth. The on-center, off-surround organization of the receptive fields also persists. P-type LGN cells in the macaque exhibit most of the properties of their retinal counterparts, including small receptive fields and color opponency.

The functional similarities between LGN cells and their retinal inputs led initially to the view that the nucleus serves merely to relay retinal signals, but it is now clear that substantial processing of these signals occurs there. An early indication of such processing was the observation that center–surround antagonism is more pronounced in geniculate than in retinal receptive fields. This enhanced antagonism probably is mediated by inhibitory GABAergic interneurons in the LGN itself and by GABAergic cells in the nearby perigeniculate nucleus, a component of the reticular nucleus of the thalamus (Figure 7.8). The inhibitory interneurons are activated by optic-tract axons (feed-forward inhibition), and the perigeniculate cells by recurrent collaterals of relay cells (feedback inhibition). The function of this complex circuitry is not understood.

Nonretinal Inputs to the LGN

In animals such as cats and monkeys, which lack an efferent projection to the retina, the LGN is the first synaptic stage of the visual pathway at which other brain systems can modulate the transmission of visual information. The potential importance of this modulation is underscored by the fact that only about 20% of the synaptic terminals in the LGN arise from retinal axons, the rest coming from nonretinal sources, including a return projection from the visual cortex, ascending projections from various brain-stem nuclei, and, as mentioned already, the perigeniculate nucleus (Figure 7.8).

The return projection from the visual cortex ends in precise retinotopic order in the geniculate laminae, and single cortico-geniculate axons may distribute terminals in more than one lamina. The projecting axons appear to excite their target cells, but inhibit neighboring neurons, presumably via geniculate interneurons or the perigeniculate nucleus. Many cells giving rise to the cortico-geniculate projection can be activated through either

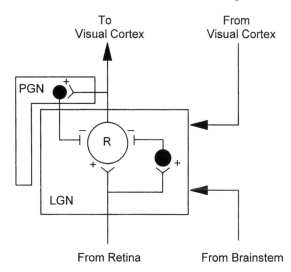

Figure 7.8. Neural circuitry of the LGN. Relay cells (R) are subject to feed-forward inhibition via intrinsic inhibitory interneurons excited by retinal afferents. Collaterals of geniculo-cortical axons activate other inhibitory cells in the perigeniculate nucleus, part of the reticular nucleus of the thalamus, creating a loop of feedback inhibition. The LGN also receives major inputs from the visual cortex and the brain stem. Black circles, inhibitory neurons.

eye. It is estimated that each LGN relay cell receives input from at least 10 cortico-geniculate fibers, in contrast to its retinal input of only one or a few optic-tract axons.

F. Schmielau and W. Singer showed that reversible inactivation of the visual cortex by cooling had a strong effect on the geometry of binocular interaction in the LGN. For example, a given cell's response to stimulation through its dominant eye might normally be facilitated by presentation of a stimulus in the center of the receptive field in the nondominant eye, but inhibited by stimulation outside this area. Cortical cooling eliminated the facilitory effect, but not the inhibition. These and other findings have led to the suggestion that the cortico-geniculate projection is important in processes involving both eyes, such as fusion of the retinal images. It has also been suggested that the feedback plays a role in selective attention to some part of the visual field. It may be fairly said, though, that the function of this projection remains a mystery.

The LGN is the target of axons from brain-stem neurons using acetyl-choline, norepinephrine, or serotonin as neurotransmitters or neuromodulators. Electrical stimulation of these inputs at their nuclei of origin modifies transmission of visual signals through the LGN. Periods of enhancement and suppression of geniculate transmission are also seen during the normal cycles of sleeping and waking. During rapid-eye-movement (REM) sleep, large electrical potentials called PGO (ponto-geniculo-occipital) waves can be recorded in the LGN and cortex. The significance of these phenomena is unknown.

Further Reading

Casagrande, V. A. (1994). A third parallel visual pathway to primate area V1. *Trends in Neurosciences* 17:305–10.

Casagrande, V. A., and Norton, T. T. (1991). Lateral geniculate nucleus: a review of its physiology and function. In *Vision and Visual Dysfunction. Vol. IV: The Neural Basis of Visual Function*, ed. A. G. Leventhal, pp. 41–84. Boca Raton: CRC Press.

Clark, W. E. Le Gros (1940). The anatomical basis of color vision. *Nature* 146: 558–9.

Cleland, B. G., and Levick, W. R. (1974). Properties of rarely encountered types of ganglion cells in the cat's retina and an overall classification. *Journal of Physiology* 240:457–92.

Schiller, P. H. (1992). The ON and OFF channels of the visual system. *Trends in Neurosciences* 15:86–92.

Schmielau, F., and Singer, W. (1977). The role of visual cortex for binocular interactions in the cat lateral geniculate nucleus. *Brain Research* 120:359–61.

Shapley, R., and Perry, V. H. (1986). Cat and monkey retinal ganglion cells and their functional roles. *Trends in Neurosciences* 9:229–35.

Sherman, S. M., and Koch, C. (1986). The control of retinogeniculate transmission in the mammalian lateral geniculate nucleus. *Experimental Brain Research* 63: 1–20.

Singer, W. (1977). Control of thalamic transmission by corticofugal and ascending reticular pathways in the visual system. *Physiological Reviews* 57:386–420.

Stone, J. (1983). *Parallel Processing in the Visual System*. New York: Plenum.

Walls, G. L. (1953). *The Lateral Geniculate Nucleus and Visual Histophysiology*. Berkeley: University of California Press.

CHAPTER 8

THE VISUAL CORTEX

Morphologic and physiologic studies have identified many regions of the cerebral cortex that are involved in vision. All of these are, in some sense, "visual cortex," but this term also has more restricted meanings. "Primary visual cortex" refers to a region of distinctive cytoarchitecture that the anatomist Brodmann designated area 17. In primates, this is the principal target of the geniculo-cortical projection. Echoing this fact, as well as its appellation of primary visual cortex, area 17 is sometimes designated V1. The term "striate cortex" arises from the presence in humans of the stria of Gennari, a prominent horizontal band in area 17 that stains heavily for myelin and is visible to the naked eye in fresh tissue. It is also called the calcarine cortex because it lies adjacent to the calcarine sulcus. Visually responsive regions outside area 17 are collectively called extrastriate areas and will be treated later in this chapter.

Effects of Lesions in Striate Cortex

Humans with complete destruction of the striate cortex on one side cease to perceive stimuli in the contralateral visual field. Partial lesions result in localized scotomata, which may be more or less "dense" depending on how much function remains. Sometimes vision is reduced to detection of motion or the presence of light. When the striate cortex and nearby regions are ablated in nonhuman primates, severe deficits are observed in tasks that presumably require visual perception. Ablation of visual cortex in other animals does not always produce such striking deficits. Cats deprived of their striate areas can execute a number of visual tasks and can navigate efficiently using visual cues. They do suffer a decrease in visual acuity and deficits on other discrimination tasks. Thus, the degree to which the visual areas of the cerebral cortex are critical in visually guided behavior, and presumably in perception, appears to vary among species.

A number of studies have reported that humans with lesions of the occipital lobe retain the ability to use retinal information for certain tasks, despite their inability to recognize this information as visual in nature. This capacity has been called "blindsight," and its existence is still somewhat controversial. The key to demonstrating these retained capacities is to give the subject no choice but to use them. For instance, a subject whose right occipital lobe has been removed surgically may be able to point rather accurately to a light in the "blind" hemifield if required to guess where the light is located. Other subjects can distinguish between two large letters, such as X and O, when they are presented in the "blind" hemifield and when the subject is required to name one or the other. The neural mechanisms subserving these preserved functions are not known, but may involve projections mediated by the superior colliculus or currently undiscovered pathways from the LGN to intact areas of the cortex.

Retinotopic Organization of the Striate Cortex

The striate cortex retains the retinotopic map of the contralateral visual field that is developed in the LGN (Figure 8.1). The boundary between the right and left hemifields of vision, usually referred to as the vertical meridian of the visual field, represents the border between area 17 and area 18. This transition region contains large numbers of neurons that project through the corpus callosum to the corresponding region in the other hemisphere and stitch together, as it were, the two halves of the visual field represented in the right and left striate cortices.

Signals of retinal origin enter the visual cortex most directly via the ascending projection from the LGN. A comparison of the geniculo-cortical projections in cat and monkey illustrates the diversity to be found in this pathway, even among mammals. The pattern in the monkey is the simplest, in that virtually all of the geniculo-cortical projection terminates in the striate cortex. Extrastriate areas receive their visual input from area 17, for the most part (Figure 8.2). In contrast, axons from the cat's LGN terminate in areas 17, 18, and 19, and the patterns of projection depend on the cell type (Figure 8.3). As noted earlier, cells of the cat's LGN generally have the properties of one of the classes of retinal ganglion cells

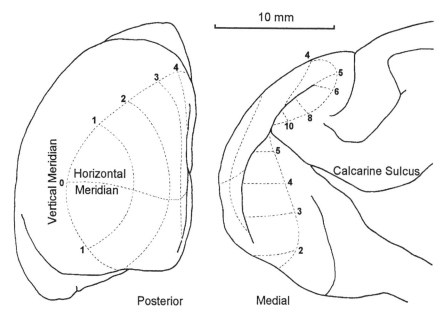

Figure 8.1. Diagrammatic representation of the central part of the retinotopic map of V1 in the squirrel monkey, estimated using field potentials evoked by small stimuli. The representation of the vertical meridian is the boundary between V1 and V2. The dotted lines are polar coordinate projections of the contralateral visual field. (Reprinted from A. Cowey: Projection of the retina onto striate and prestriate cortex in the squirrel monkey, *Saimiri sciureus. Journal of Neurophysiol*ogy 27:366–93, 1964, with permission of the American Physiological Society.)

and are also called W, X, or Y cells. In the geniculo-cortical projection, X cells of the laminated LGN project to area 17, and Y cells of these laminae send branches to areas 17 and 18. Y cells of the MIN project to area 18 and the lateral suprasylvian cortex. W cells of the C laminae project to areas 17, 18, and 19.

Major Types of Neuronal Cells in the Striate Cortex

Geniculate and other afferents to the cortex form the inputs to complex circuits composed of cortical neurons and their projections to targets both inside and outside the cortex. Three basic morphologic types of neurons have been identified in the striate cortex, each exhibiting several subclasses or varieties. The dendrites of spiny stellate cells have a radiating or star-shaped form and are covered with short cytoplasmic excrescences called spines (Figure 8.4A). The dendrites of smooth stellate cells are devoid of

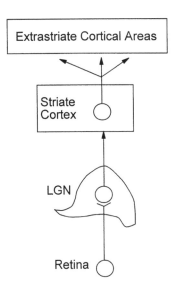

Figure 8.2. Diagram of primate pattern of geniculo-cortical projection.

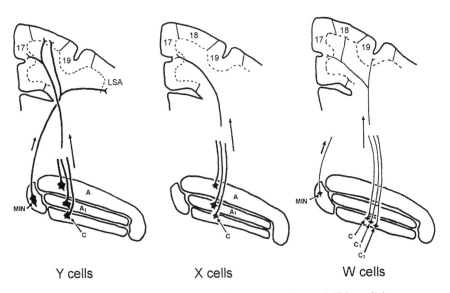

Y cells   X cells   W cells

Figure 8.3. Projection of the LGN to the cerebral cortex in the cat. MIN, medial intralaminar nucleus; LSA, lateral suprasylvian area. (Reprinted from J. Stone: *Parallel Processing in the Visual System*. Copyright 1983, with permission of Plenum Publishing Corporation.)

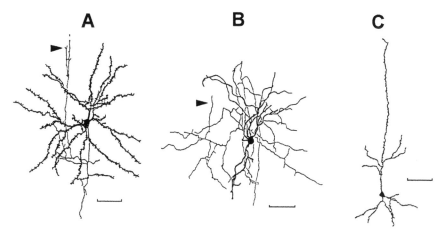

Figure 8.4. Cell types in the striate cortex. (A) Spiny stellate cell from a kitten aged about 5 weeks. [Reprinted from J. S. Lund, G. H. Henry, C. L. MacQueen, and A. R. Harvey: Anatomical organization of the primary visual cortex (area 17) of the cat. A comparison with area 17 of the macaque monkey. *Journal of Comparative Neurology* 184:599–618, 1979, with permission of Wiley-Liss, Inc., a subsidiary of John Wiley & Sons.] (B) Aspinous stellate cell from adult macaque. [Reprinted from J. S. Lund: Organization of neurons in the visual cortex, area 17, of the monkey (*Macaca mulatta*). *Journal of Comparative Neurology* 147:455–96, 1973, with permission of Wiley-Liss, Inc., a subsidiary of John Wiley & Sons.] (C) Pyramidal cell from adult macaque. [Reprinted from J. S. Lund, R. G. Boothe, and R. D. Lund: Development of neurons in the visual cortex (area 17) of the monkey (*Macaca nemestrina*): A Golgi study from fetal day 127 to postnatal maturity. *Journal of Comparative Neurology* 176:149–88, 1979, with permission of Wiley-Liss, Inc., a subsidiary of John Wiley & Sons.] The bar is 50 μm in each panel. Arrowheads mark recurrent and locally arborizing axon collaterals.

spines (Figure 8.4B). Many smooth stellate cells contain GABA and are believed to be inhibitory neurons acting within the cortex itself. Pyramidal cells constitute the other major cell type in the striate cortex and are named for their pyramid-shaped cell bodies. Spines encrust a single ascending apical dendrite of varying length and several basal dendrites (Figure 8.4C).

The axons of pyramidal cells often have ascending collaterals that tend to remain close to the cells' apical dendrites, giving a columnar character to the local circuitry. This is mirrored in the tendency of afferents from the LGN and elsewhere representing the same part of the visual field to restrict their terminals to a small cylindrical volume of cortex. More will be said about this later, but it is important to note that pyramidal cell axons or their collaterals may also extend laterally in a given lamina and are capable of mediating interactions between points in the striate cortex several millimeters apart.

Cortical Microcircuitry

The striate cortex contains a variety of neural circuits linked to other cortical areas, to subcortical structures, and to each other. A useful guide to the identity and nature of the circuits is provided by the disposition of cortical cells, which gives a layered appearance to area 17, as it does to other regions of the cerebral cortex (Figure 8.5). Anatomists have devised numbering systems for the layers based on cell size and other morphologic characteristics, and current practice is to distinguish six main layers, with layer 1 adjacent to the pia, and layer 6 bounded by the white matter. Because the cells in part of layer 4 of area 17 generally have small cell bodies and are densely packed, this zone is sometimes referred to as the granular layer. The more superficial layers 1–3 are called supragranular, and the deeper layers 5 and 6 infragranular. The main laminae are also designated by Roman numerals I–VI, as in Figure 8.5. For consistency's sake, and to avoid potentially confusing expressions such as "layer IV in V1," this book will identify the main cortical layers using Arabic numerals.

Anatomists also distinguish sublaminae in several of the main cortical layers. Thus, the numbering system of Figure 8.5 distinguishes four sublaminae in layer 4. Other anatomists believe that layer 3 should incorporate what in Figure 8.5 are labeled as sublaminae IVA and IVB, leaving only two sublaminae in layer 4 (Figure 8.6). The systems of laminar designations continue to evolve as more is learned about the circuitry in which the various cortical neurons participate.

LGN afferents project to the various laminae in the striate cortex in patterns that vary from species to species and among classes of afferent fibers. In all species, the majority of geniculate axons terminate about midway through the thickness of area 17 (Figure 8.6). Afferents of a given origin may be further segregated within the sublaminae of the principal layers. Thus, the magnocellular LGN neurons of primates project to layer 4α, and the parvocellular neurons to layer 4ß, but they also give off collaterals in layer 6 (Figure 8.6). The putative koniocellular pathway terminates in layers 3B and 1. In layer 3B, the terminals of this projection are concentrated in small regions that have high levels of cytochrome oxidase, an enzyme associated with structures having intense metabolic activity (dotted oval in Figure 8.6). These zones rich in cytochrome oxidase are sometimes referred to as "blobs," from their appearance in appropriately stained sections of the striate cortex. Extrastriate cortical areas send return projections to area 17, with terminations in many laminae. The general pattern

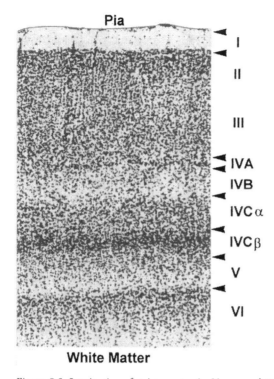

Pia

I

II

III

IVA

IVB

IVC α

IVC β

V

VI

White Matter

Figure 8.5. Lamination of striate cortex in *Macaca mulatta*. Cytoarchitecture as seen in a section stained for Nissl substance. [Reprinted from J. S. Lund: Organization of neurons in the visual cortex, area 17, of the monkey (*Macaca mulatta*). *Journal of Comparative Neurology* 147:455–96, 1973, with permission of Wiley-Liss, Inc., a subsidiary of John Wiley & Sons.]

in the cat is remarkably similar. X- and Y-type LGN axons terminate principally in layer 4, but also contribute collaterals to layer 6. W cells terminate mainly in layer 1, but distribute collaterals to layers 3 and 5.

Cells in a given lamina may participate in circuits that involve other laminae as well as structures outside the striate cortex. As an example, pyramidal cells in layer 5 have apical dendrites that may extend all the way to layer 1 and are thus positioned to be influenced from all the overlying layers (Figure 8.6, left). These same cells send a major projection to the superior colliculus and also emit axon collaterals that arborize in the supragranular layers. A similar pattern is seen in those layer-6 pyramidal cells sending axons back to the LGN. Cells in supragranular layers 2 and 3 provide the major efferent projections to extrastriate cortex and distribute local collaterals to other cortical layers. Their apical dendrites extend to

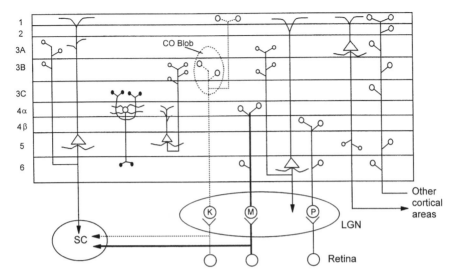

Figure 8.6. Cortical microcircuitry in area V1 of macaque monkey. Pyramidal cells are shown with triangular cell bodies. The cell with a circular black soma is an inhibitory stellate cell making local contacts (small filled circles). Small open circles are excitatory contacts. SC, superior colliculus; LGN, lateral geniculate nucleus; K, koniocellular; M, magnocellular; P, parvocellular; CO, cytochrome oxidase. Not all inputs to the striate cortex are illustrated here. Note the parallel projection of the K and M pathways to both cortex and SC. [Adapted from V. A. Casagrande: A third visual pathway to primate area V1. *Trends in Neurosciences* 17: 305–10, 1944, and J. S. Lund, G. H. Henry, C. L. MacQueen, and A. R. Harvey: Anatomical organization of the primary visual cortex (area 17) of the cat. A comparison with area 17 of the macaque monkey. *Journal of Comparative Neurology* 184: 599–618, 1979.]

layer 1. Stellate cells and some pyramidal cells distribute their axonal terminals entirely within the cortex and function as inhibitory or excitatory local-circuit neurons (Figure 8.6).

Binocularity and Ocular Dominance in the Striate Cortex

One striking feature of cortical cells is that, in contrast to the lateral geniculate neurons providing their input, the cortical cells usually respond to stimulation of either eye, and therefore they have receptive fields on both retinas. However, the early stages of cortical processing do not fully eliminate the distinction between signals arising in the left and right eyes. Various tracer studies and staining techniques have revealed that the ter-

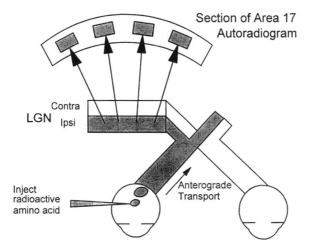

Figure 8.7. Trans-synaptic labeling of ocular-dominance regions in the striate cortex.

minals from the monocular LGN laminae occupy alternating bands in layer 4. In the experiment schematized in Figure 8.7, a radioactive amino acid is injected into one eye. Taken up by the ganglion cells, the tracer moves by anterograde axonal transport to the LGN, where it migrates from the axon terminals to nearby postsynaptic cells in the target lamina. These cells transport the tracer to the cortex, where it produces a patchy labeling in layer 4. When the pattern of these alternating regions is reconstructed for all of layer 4, the zones appear as branching stripes that meander across the cortex to end at the boundary between areas 17 and 18.

Not surprisingly, cells of layer 4 tend to be driven predominantly, and sometimes exclusively, from one eye or the other. If an electrode samples cells in a penetration that is normal to the surface of the cortex, most of the cells it encounters respond best to stimulation of the eye represented in the patch of layer 4 traversed by the electrode. These vertically oriented regions of similar ocular preference were at first thought to be columnar in shape and were called ocular-dominance columns. This terminology is still used, although it is now known that the regions are shaped more like slabs than columns. If the recording electrode traverses the cortex parallel to the cortical surface and across the slabs, the ocular dominance of the cells oscillates from one eye to the other in a continuous fashion.

D. H. Hubel and T. N. Wiesel introduced the practice of classifying cells according to the degree to which their responses are dominated by one eye or the other. Figure 8.8 illustrates a typical ocular-dominance histogram for a large sample of cortical neurons of the cat. The exact shape of such a histogram depends on which layers are sampled, because cells in layer 4 tend to lie at the extremes of the distribution (categories 1 and 7), and those in the supragranular and infragranular layers in the intermediate categories.

It is unknown why there is continuing partial spatial segregation in the cortex of signals originating in the left and right eyes. A reasonable guess might be that fusion of two slightly different retinal images and the extraction of stereoscopic distance information depend on preserving some distinction between left and right eye signals at the cortical level. Ocular-dominance columns are either absent or poorly defined in some animals with binocular visual fields, such as tree shrews, certain New World monkeys, lagomorphs, rodents, and ungulates, but it is not known to what extent stereoscopic vision suffers as a consequence of this.

Visual Experience and the Development of Ocular Dominance in the Striate Cortex

Ocular-dominance columns are not present in newborn kittens, but develop during the first few weeks of life after the lids open and the ocular media become clear. At birth, the geniculate afferents representing the two eyes intermingle extensively in layer 4. In a series of pioneering studies, Wiesel and Hubel demonstrated that visual stimulation of both eyes is essential for segregation of the LGN afferents, which is the basis for the ocular-dominance columns. If the lids of one eye are sutured together, depriving that eye of pattern stimulation for a period of weeks, the majority of neurons in striate cortex recorded later respond only to stimulation through the open eye. Also, the anatomic markers of ocular dominance show parallel effects. The cortical stripes labeled by transneuronal transport of radioactive amino acids from the deprived eye (Figure 8.7) become very thin, and neurons in the geniculate layers representing the deprived eye undergo changes resembling atrophy (see Figure 7.2). It is as if the deprived eye were disconnected from the brain. These changes are accompanied by behavioral effects indicating that the sensitivity and acuity of the deprived eye are greatly reduced, a condition known as amblyopia. Comparable findings have been reported for primates.

A large body of experimental evidence indicates that the ocular-dominance columns normally form as a result of competition for cortical synaptic space by the LGN afferents representing the two eyes. This competition is dependent on the level and timing of neural activity in the two monocular pathways, and normally its outcome is determined during a limited window of time in the animal's life, the so-called critical period (4–12 weeks in cats, 0–8 weeks in monkeys). When one eye is deprived

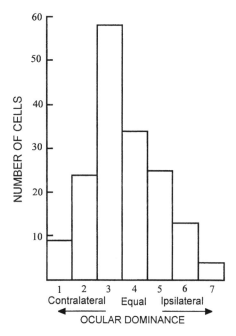

Figure 8.8. Ocular-dominance histogram for a sample of neurons in striate cortex of an adult cat. (Reprinted from D. H. Hubel and T. N. Wiesel: Binocular interaction in striate cortex of kittens raised with artificial squint. *Journal of Neurophysiology* 28:1041–59, 1965, with permission of the American Physiological Society.)

of patterned stimulation and becomes less active, its cortical territory is taken over by afferents from the open, stimulated eye.

If at some point during the critical period the open eye is occluded and the previously deprived eye is exposed to patterned stimulation, the effects on ocular dominance can be reversed. The degree of reversal depends on a number of factors, including the duration of deprivation and the age at which the manipulations occur. These phenomena have provided an experimental model that is widely used in studies of the nature of neural plasticity. The ocular-dominance shift induced by monocular deprivation is an example of activity-dependent reorganization of neural tissue, which may be related to the mechanisms of memory and learning.

The amblyopia induced by monocular deprivation in experimental animals is reminiscent of that observed in humans whose early visual experience is disturbed by conditions that disrupt normal binocular vision, such as congenital cataract or abnormal ocular alignment. Prompt intervention during the early years of life can prevent or diminish the loss of vision resulting from these conditions.

Receptive Fields of Neurons in the Striate Cortex

The center–surround organization characteristic of the receptive fields of retinal and LGN cells undergoes a major transformation at the cortical level. Although the receptive fields of some cells in layer 4 retain a center–surround configuration, those of most cortical neurons are very different. Two major categories of cortical receptive fields were identified by Hubel and Wiesel, and the names given to these fields and the cells that exhibit them continue to be used by most investigators (Figure 8.9). In simple receptive fields, on areas and off areas remain spatially separate, but are elongated and aligned next to one another in various combinations. On zones and off zones are superimposed in complex receptive fields, much as they are in some specialized receptive fields of the retina.

Simple cells are optimally excited by oriented line segments or bars that match the contrast pattern of the receptive field. For example, a cell whose receptive field has a central on strip flanked by two off strips is maximally excited by a light bar covering the central strip (Figure 8.9). The optimal orientation of this bar is predictable from the disposition of on areas and off areas in the receptive field. As one rotates the light bar, it encroaches on off areas, evoking an inhibitory influence that reduces the response of the cell (Figure 8.9, top right). Complex cells, like simple cells, respond best to oriented bars or edges, but their preferred orientations are not predictable from the disposition of on zones and off zones within the receptive fields. The location of the bar or edge in its receptive field is critical for the simple cell, but not for the complex cell (Figure 8.9, left).

Simple cells and complex cells often exhibit directional selectivity, responding most vigorously to stimulus motion in a particular direction, and giving reduced responses to movements in other directions. The responses of both simple and complex cells often can be inhibited by extending a stimulus beyond the region yielding on responses and off responses to flashed spots or bars. This central region is sometimes referred to as the "classical receptive field." Cells exhibiting these inhibitory flanks or surrounds were originally believed to constitute a separate functional class, called hypercomplex, but that notion has been largely abandoned. Flanking inhibition appears to be a variable property of both simple and complex cells.

Microelectrode techniques that allow an investigator to classify the receptive field of a cell and then inject the cell with a substance that permits its visualization have failed to reveal a strict correlation between physiologic and morphologic types of cortical neurons. Some stellate cells have complex receptive fields, and others simple receptive fields. Although pyramidal cells tend to have complex receptive fields, there are exceptions.

Simple Cell

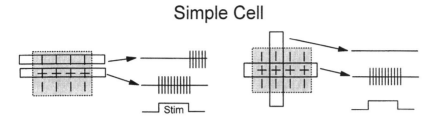

Complex Cell

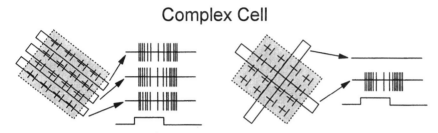

Figure 8.9. Schematic examples of simple (top) and complex (bottom) cortical receptive fields. The on areas (plus signs) and off areas (minus signs) are spatially separate in the receptive fields of simple cells, and superimposed in complex cells. The position of the stimulus in the receptive field is critical for the simple cell, but not for the complex cell (left). Changing the orientation of the elongated stimulus from its optimum reduces the responses of both kinds of cells (right).

The Role of Taxonomy in the Study of Cortical Neurons

It is useful at this point to consider briefly the significance of cell classification per se in the analysis of a structure such as the visual cortex. These considerations apply as well to other parts of the visual system, including the retina and the LGN. An enormous amount of experimental and theoretical effort has been devoted to refining the classification schemes applied to cortical neurons based on their physiologic and morphologic properties. These efforts continue, in the expectation that a cell's properties will reveal something about its functional role in vision. It does not follow, though, that cells with identical properties have identical roles in vision. For example, cells with the same morphologic and physiologic characteristics may participate in circuits mediating distinct visual processes, in the same way that a particular kind of transistor can be a component in a variety of electronic circuits. This last point recalls the observation made earlier that the axons of retinal Y cells distribute terminals to several central nuclei, each of which may exploit some characteristics of the cell's responses, but not necessarily all of them.

In their emphasis on the single cell, classification schemes generally tend to ignore the fact that a given stimulus affects countless neurons spread over substantial areas of the visual cortex and that the features of this distribution of activity may be as important in encoding the stimulus as the response properties of the individual neurons themselves. It is worth keeping this in mind as we later discuss the way in which cortical neurons are "tuned" to various aspects of a stimulus.

As emphasized by J. Stone, classification schemes that purport to identify functional classes of neurons based on their physiologic and morphologic properties are hypotheses that are subject to refinement and even rejection as knowledge accumulates. A good example of refinement is the continuing reclassification of some retinal W cells into more homogeneous functional groupings on the basis of their morphologies, projections, and receptive-field properties. The abandonment of the hypercomplex classification of cortical neurons is an instance in which experimental observations reduced the number of hypothetical functional groups. Some classification schemes may be airtight, in that they assign all neurons to one or another class, but this does not guarantee their usefulness in understanding how a given neuron functions in vision.

The Neural Substrates of Receptive Fields in Visual Cortex

The response properties of neurons in visual cortex arise ultimately from the circuits that connect the cells to the retina and other parts of the brain. The first attempt to account for the differences between simple and complex cells was that of Hubel and Wiesel, who proposed what is known as the hierarchical or serial model. According to this idea, simple cells combine the inputs of an array of LGN neurons of one type (on-center or off-center) whose receptive fields are distributed along a straight line in visual space. Thus, a convergent array of on-center LGN cells would give rise to a simple receptive field with a central on strip flanked by off strips. Simple cells were thought to represent the first stage of cortical processing, a notion supported by the finding that these cells tended to occur most often in layers 4 and 6, which receive direct retinal projections. Complex cells were assumed to acquire their receptive fields by summing the inputs of several simple cells with similar orientation preferences. This would explain why all points in a complex receptive field yield both on and off responses and why complex cells also prefer borders or bars with a particular orientation, but are indifferent to the position of the stimulus within the receptive field. In its earlier formulation, the hierarchical model was extended to include hypercomplex cells, which were thought to result from the summation of inputs from an array of complex cells. It is this putative hierarchical arrangement that is implied in the terms "simple," "complex," and "hypercomplex."

Although the hierarchical model is consistent with many properties of simple and complex cells, various findings indicate that cortical connectivity is considerably more complex than is implied by the model. For example, it is known that both simple and complex cells can receive monosynaptic input from the LGN. Complex cells readily respond to stimuli moving at velocities greater than those to which the majority of simple cells are sensitive. The directional selectivity of complex cells also cannot be predicted from the distribution of on areas and off areas alone, which implies additional intracortical processing, presumably involving inhibitory interneurons. From these and other observations it would appear that more than just serial connectivity is involved in constructing the receptive fields of neurons of the visual cortex. Thus, simple cells may indeed provide input to complex cells, but both types also appear to be activated in parallel by geniculate inputs and to be subject to additional synaptic modulation by intracortical circuitry.

Orientation Preferences of Neurons in the Visual Cortex

Perhaps the most striking feature of cortical neurons discovered by Hubel and Wiesel is their preference for elongated stimuli having a particular orientation (Figure 8.9). The presence of this feature poses formidable problems of circuit analysis and interpretation. The basic observation is that when a bar or edge is presented in the receptive field of a cortical cell, the cell's response is modulated as a function of the orientation of the stimulus. That some orientations yield more vigorous responses than others is said to reflect the orientation tuning of the cell. Examples of orientation-tuning curves for two simple cells are shown in Figure 8.10. Observe that the cells do not respond to just one orientation, but discharge most vigorously to a preferred orientation, which can be identified with greater or lesser precision depending on the variability of the cell's responses. The tuning curves for the two cells also differ in their sharpness or selectivity. Orientation selectivity is often expressed quantitatively as the half-width at half-height of the tuning curve, the steepness of the curve's shoulders, or some other comparable measure.

If a recording electrode descends through the cortical layers normal to the surface, the cells encountered tend to prefer the same stimulus orientation. This observation gave rise to the notion that the cortex is organized into orientation columns that run from white matter to pia. When the electrode passes diagonally across the cortical thickness or parallel to the

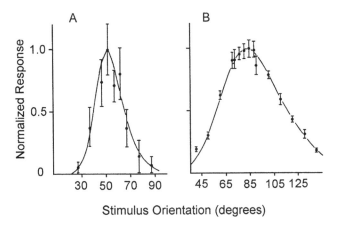

Figure 8.10. Orientation tuning curves for two simple cells. The magnitudes of the cells' responses were measured as a moving bar traversed the receptive field at different orientations. These are means of 10 presentations of the moving bar. Vertical bars represent standard errors. (Reprinted, with permission, from P. Heggelund and K. Albus: Response variability and orientation discrimination of single cells in striate cortex of cat. *Experimental Brain Research* 32:197–212. Copyright 1978, Springer-Verlag.)

cortical surface in both cat and monkey, the preferred orientations of the cells often rotate systematically through 180° over a distance of about 1 mm, and the cycle is then repeated (Figure 8.11). Dislocations are sometimes encountered, at which the direction of rotation reverses, or a jump occurs in the preferred angle. These observations imply that the orientation tuning of cortical cells is governed by some mechanism that bestows a common preference on columns of cells oriented normal to the surface and is orderly and piecewise periodic across the cortex.

Efforts to determine the spatial dispositions and sizes of orientation columns have taken several forms. It was first believed, on the basis of electrophysiologic mapping studies, that the columns were several hundred micrometers in width, but subsequent work indicated that shifts in preferred orientation could be detected when an electrode was advanced no more than 20 μm. This is about the soma diameter of a cortical pyramidal neuron, suggesting that the columns are about one cell thick. Another way of interpreting these findings is that some mechanism produces an "orientation field" in which the cortical cells reside and that varies across the cortex and is sampled by the cells located at any given position within it. The field influences a given cell most strongly at the position of the soma, which determines the preferred orientation of the cell. Increasingly

Preferred
Orientation   Microelectrode track

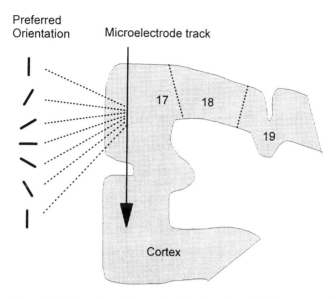

Figure 8.11. Rotation of the preferred orientations of cells encountered in a schematic microelectrode penetration parallel to the surface of area 17 in the cat. The
preferred orientation is indicated by the line segments to the left of this diagram
of a coronal section.

more distant parts of the field, representing different orientations, have
diminishing influences on the cell.

Hubel and Wiesel observed that a cortical patch containing a full 180°
of orientation columns was about the same size as that spanned by two
ocular-dominance columns. They suggested that this patch, which is between 1 and 2 mm in diameter in macaque striate cortex, represents a
functional cortical module, because it contains all the machinery needed
to analyze the region of visual space that it represents. They noted that
such a module, which has sometimes been called a hypercolumn, has rather
arbitrary boundaries; where it ends depends on which orientation or ocular-
dominance column is chosen as its beginning. According to this concept
of functional cortical architecture, the striate cortex is tiled with hypercolumns, each analyzing adjacent regions of visual space.

Two methods have been employed to visualize the sizes and distributions of orientation columns. In the first, radioactive 2-deoxy-D-glucose
(2DG), an unmetabolizable analogue of glucose, is injected intravenously
into an animal stimulated continuously with a grating of a particular orientation. The 2DG is taken up by active elements that can then be visualized in autoradiographs of the brain tissue. When a grating is pre-

sented repeatedly at a given orientation, the labeled regions have the form of spots or bands and occupy about half of the volume of the cortex. This is not surprising, because, as is evident from the orientation-tuning curves, cells respond to a range of orientations, not just to stimuli at the preferred orientation. Thus, an oriented stimulus may be expected to activate some cells maximally, and neighboring cells less intensely. A technical problem with 2DG studies of this type is that the metabolic tag tends to label areas with high spontaneous activity, such as the cytochrome oxidase blobs mentioned earlier, and cannot distinguish between orientation-selective regions and those activated by any stimulus regardless of its orientation.

The second method used to map orientation columns depends on changes in the optical properties of active neural tissue. In one version of this technique, the cortex is soaked with a dye that absorbs more or less light of a particular wavelength as the membrane potentials of the cortical cells vary. The absorption patterns, presumably reflecting patterns of neural activity, are recorded by special optical equipment while stimulus gratings are presented at various orientations (Figure 8.12). A variation on this approach dispenses with dyes and measures intrinsic light scatter in the tissue during stimulation, perhaps due to local changes in blood flow. The success of both methods depends on presenting a stimulus of one orientation followed by a stimulus at the orthogonal orientation, and then subtracting one activity distribution from the other. This has the effect of highlighting regions that respond preferentially to the two orthogonal orientations and canceling signals from areas that respond equally well to both. Thus, the subtraction method is well suited to mapping preferred orientations, but it underestimates the area activated by a particular orientation.

Figure 8.13 summarizes the results of an experiment by G. G. Blasdel in which responses to a series of orthogonal pairs of orientations were analyzed to produce a spatial map of orientation preferences in a small region of cortex. When patterns were subtracted from each other, regions responding preferentially to a particular orientation could be identified. The swirls of oriented line segments in this figure represent the preferred orientations of neighboring neurons, the lengths of the lines reflecting the degree of selectivity. Black dots and squiggles correspond to loci where orientation preferences change rapidly over short distances, either because of a jump in the preferred orientation or because of a sudden reversal in the local sequence. At some of these loci the preferred orientations are arranged like pinwheels.

The neural mechanisms responsible for orientation preference are not known. It has been suggested that the process begins in the retina, with ganglion cells that respond to one orientation slightly more vigorously

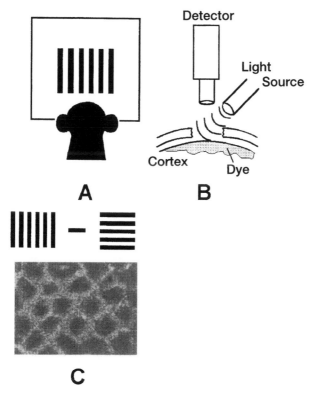

Figure 8.12. Optical measurement of orientation columns. (A) The animal views a screen on which are presented gratings of different orientations. (B) Specialized video detectors measure changes in the absorption properties of a voltage-sensitive dye that has been superfused on the cortex. (C) Schematic illustration of map resulting when voltage patterns produced by drifting gratings of orthogonal orientations have been subtracted from each other, so that the dark areas and light areas correspond to regions most active in response to the orthogonal orientations.

than to others. According to the hierarchical scheme of Hubel and Wiesel, orientation tuning is due to the geometry of geniculate inputs to cortical simple cells, which then pass on their preferred orientations to other cells. Local application of bicuculline, a $GABA_A$-receptor blocker, eliminates or reduces orientation tuning in nearby cortical neurons, suggesting that intracortical inhibitory circuitry is critical for this phenomenon, but the issue remains unsettled. Elucidation of the neural basis of orientation tuning remains one of the central problems of visual neuroscience.

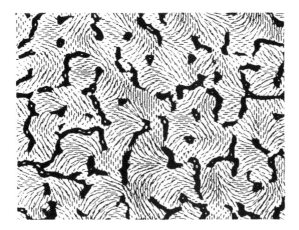

Figure 8.13. A map of preferred orientations in the striate cortex of the macaque monkey. The field covers an area of 3 x 4 mm. Optical recording methods registered patterns of activity evoked by a range of orientations. (From G. G. Blasdel: Orientation selectivity, preference and continuity in monkey striate cortex. *Journal of Neuroscience* 12:3139–61, 1992, with permission of the Society for Neuroscience.)

What Is the Function of Orientation Tuning?

The shortest answer to this question is that no one knows. The discovery of orientation tuning came at a time when it was widely believed that single cells with specific stimulus preferences were labeled lines, meaning that a cell's discharge signaled unambiguously the presence of the stimulus feature to which that cell was most responsive. This view is an extension of Müller's "law of specific nerve energies" to the single-cell level. Müller argued that activation of the optic nerve, for instance, always resulted in a visual perception, regardless of how the nerve was excited. The most extreme application of Müller's law holds that the discharge of some neurons has a fixed significance for perception and that the features encoded are the ordinary elements of perception, such as lines, colors, and so forth. Neurons whose discharge is thought to signify a particular aspect of a stimulus are sometimes referred to as feature detectors. These ideas are captured in the facetious notion of the "grandmother cell," a cell whose activity would signify the presence of one's grandmother.

At the time of their discovery, then, it was natural to relate the presence of cells with orientation tuning to the perception of oriented lines and edges, such as occur commonly in the visual environment. There are, however, several difficulties with this idea that encourage a skeptical view of it. Orientation-tuning curves are relatively broad, and the cells' responses are modulated by other factors such as stimulus contrast and the direction and speed of motion. Some orientation-tuned cells are more sensitive to small moving spots than to oriented line segments. This means that a single orientation-tuned neuron can fire with comparable vigor to orientations that differ widely or even to nonoriented stimuli. In short, the discharge rate of such a cell is an ambiguous signal of stimulus orientation.

The temptation to leap from the stimulus preferences of single neurons to elements of perception is arguably a consequence of the technical advances that permitted recordings of the activities of single neurons. When observing the activity of a single cell that responds vigorously to a given stimulus, it is easy to forget that there are countless other neurons responding to the same stimulus and that they also may be involved in its coding. With respect to orientation, it is worth noting that the spatial distributions of cortical cells responding to the letters X and Y must be different, and that difference, rather than the preferred orientations of the active neurons, may be the basis of our ability to distinguish between the two letters.

Extrastriate Visual Cortex

As noted at the beginning of this chapter, visually responsive cells are found outside area 17 in regions referred to collectively as extrastriate visual cortex. These areas are usually interconnected with striate cortex and with each other by a system of reciprocal projections, both direct and indirect. In the cat, certain extrastriate areas receive projections directly from the LGN (Figure 8.4). Figure 8.14 shows the locations of several identified extrastriate visual areas in the primate. Some of these have unique designations, such as the middle temporal area (MT), and others are labeled V2, V3, V4, and so forth, by analogy with V1.

An area of extrastriate visual cortex is usually assumed to be a functional unit if it exhibits a homogeneous pattern of afferent and efferent connections, uniformity in the properties of its cells, and the presence of a single retinotopic map. Cytoarchitectural and myeloarchitectural features tend to be less reliable guides to the boundaries of functional entities in extrastriate cortex than in area 17 and nearby regions. Not all tentatively identified areas satisfy all of these criteria, and the parceling of extrastriate cortex changes as new information is acquired. Recent technical developments in brain imaging have permitted studies of the human brain during the performance of visual and other tasks. These methods, most of which measure changes in regional blood flow that presumably mirror neuronal activity, hold great promise for mapping the extrastriate areas of the human brain and assessing their roles in vision.

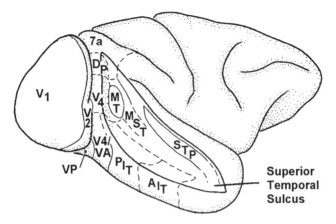

Figure 8.14. Visual areas outside area 17 or V1 in the macaque. The superior temporal sulcus has been opened up to reveal areas such as MT concealed within it. Areas buried in other sulci are not shown in this diagram. (Adapted from J. H. R. Maunsell and W. T. Newsome: Visual processing in monkey extrastriate cortex. *Annual Review of Neuroscience* 10:363–401, 1987, with permission of Annual Reviews, Inc.)

The projection from area 17 to area 18 offers a good example of why it is believed that major transformations of the encoded visual image occur at early stages of cortical processing. The retinotopic map of area 18 in the cat is highly compressed relative to that in area 17, and the upper and lower visual fields are not represented contiguously over much of the map. Also, in primates, the patterns of cytochrome oxidase staining differ significantly in the two areas: Labeling is punctate or blob-like in area 17, but distributed in stripes in area 18. A complex pattern of connections links the so-called blob and interblob regions of area 17 to the cytochrome oxidase stripes and interstripes of area 18. Information arriving by way of the P and M pathways is distributed and combined in a complex manner.

The projections from V1 to extrastriate cortex are consistent with a proposal that visual information flows in two major streams (Figure 8.15). One of these, the parietal stream, is thought to be involved in the processing of spatial information and reaches the parietal lobe via certain areas in the superior temporal sulcus. The temporal stream is directed toward the inferior part of the temporal lobe and is believed to be concerned with object recognition and color perception. Extensive clinical observations in humans have long indicated that lesions in the parietal lobe tend to disturb perceptions of spatial relationships, whereas temporal-lobe lesions can interfere with memory for objects and faces. A growing body of work in

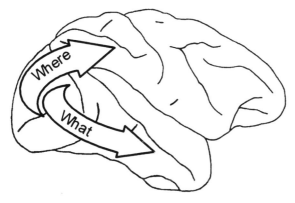

Figure 8.15. The parietal and temporal streams from V1 and V2. This cartoon highlights the idea that the parietal stream is concerned with spatial localization, and the temporal stream with object identification. (Adapted from M. Mishkin, L. G. Ungerleider, and K. A. Macko: Object vision and spatial vision: two cortical pathways. *Trends in Neurosciences* 6:414–17, 1983, with permission of Elsevier Trends Journals.)

experimental animals generally supports such a functional specialization in these two regions of the cortex.

Area MT (Figure 8.14), one of the most extensively studied of the extrastriate visual areas, offers a good example of a component of the putative parietal pathway. This area receives direct inputs from V1 and V2 and projects, in turn, to other structures connected to the parietal lobe. Cells in MT have large receptive fields and are highly selective for movement direction. The cells are binocular, but are not tuned to orientation. Lesions in this area temporarily impair a monkey's ability to discriminate movement direction in the part of the visual field represented at the lesion site. When a monkey views a field of randomly distributed moving dots, of which only a small fraction is moving in the same direction, and is required to identify the direction of this coherent motion with an appropriately directed eye movement, the discharge of cells in MT provides an estimate of stimulus direction as accurate as the behavior of the monkey. Focal electrical stimulation in MT biases the choices made by the monkey in favor of the preferred direction of the cells near the stimulating electrode. Taken together, these findings suggest that MT plays a critical role in the perception of motion and is relatively unconcerned with the form of the moving object.

In contrast, neurons in the inferior temporal cortex are influenced by both the M and P pathways and often exhibit preferences for stimuli of particular colors and shapes. Lesions of the temporal cortex can disrupt object discriminations based on color, shape, and brightness, but have little or no effect on movement perception or global spatial discriminations. Such lesions also interfere with the performance of visual memory tasks.

A cautionary note is provided by the finding that lesions in both the parietal and temporal cortices produce transient deficits, indicating that functions are more widely distributed than would be implied by the two-stream model, or that other areas are capable of assuming functions once mediated by the lesioned area. Thus, the idea of two separate streams of visual processing, one addressing the "what" and the other the "where" of an object (Figure 8.15), serves as a useful rule of thumb, but clearly oversimplifies the brain's strategy for encoding these aspects of the visual scene.

Further Reading

Barlow, H. B. (1972). Single units and sensation: a neuron doctrine for perceptual psychology. *Perception* 1:371–94.

Blasdel, G. G. (1992). Orientation selectivity, preference and continuity in monkey striate cortex. *Journal of Neuroscience* 12:3139–61.

Bonhoeffer, T., and Grinvald, A. (1991). Iso-orientation domains in cat visual cortex are arranged in pinwheel-like patterns. *Nature* 353:429–31.

Britten, K. H., Shadlen, M. N., Newsome, W. T., and Movshon, J. A. (1992). The analysis of visual motion: a comparison of neuronal and psychophysical performance. *Journal of Neuroscience* 12:4745–65.

Casagrande, V. A. (1994). A third visual pathway to primate area V1. *Trends in Neurosciences* 17:305–10.

Cowey, A., and Stoerig, P. (1991). The neurobiology of blindsight. *Trends in Neurosciences* 14:140–5.

Hubel, D. H. (1988). *Eye, Brain, and Vision.* New York: Scientific American Library.

Hubel, D. H., and Wiesel, T. N. (1977). Ferrier lecture: functional architecture of macaque monkey visual cortex. *Proceedings of the Royal Society of London* 198: 1–59.

Livingstone, M. S., and Hubel, D. H. (1984). Anatomy and physiology of a color system in the primate visual cortex. *Journal of Neuroscience* 4:309–56.

Lund, J. S., Henry, G. H., MacQueen, C. L., and Harvey, A. R. (1979). Anatomical organization of the primary visual cortex (area 17) of the cat. A comparison with area 17 of the macaque monkey. *Journal of Comparative Neurology* 184: 599–618.

Maunsell, J. H. R., and Newsome, W. T. (1987). Visual processing in monkey extrastriate cortex. *Annual Review of Neuroscience* 10:363–401.

Merigan, W. H., and Maunsell, J. H. R. (1993). How parallel are the primate visual pathways? *Annual Review of Neuroscience* 16:369–402.

Mishkin, M., Ungerleider, L. G., and Macko, K. A. (1983). Object vision and spatial vision: two cortical pathways. *Trends in Neurosciences* 6:414–17.

Stone, J. (1983). *Parallel Processing in the Visual System.* New York: Plenum.

Wiesel, T. N. (1982). Postnatal development of the visual cortex and influence of environment (Nobel lecture). *Nature* 299:583–91.

PART III

SPECIAL TOPICS IN VISION

CHAPTER 9

SPATIAL RESOLUTION IN VISION

The capacity of a visual system to resolve fine spatial detail depends on several factors, some associated with the stimulus object, others with the eye, and still others with the central visual pathways. Sensitivity to spatial detail is commonly called acuity, but it is important to remember that this word is applied to several different performance measures. One reads, for example, of minimum separable acuity, grating acuity, vernier acuity, and stereoscopic acuity. The neural mechanisms that mediate these discriminative capacities are not necessarily all the same, despite the fact that the same word, "acuity," is used for them. It should also be kept in mind that these measurements usually reflect performance at the extreme limit of some functional capacity, rather like determinations of the absolute threshold for detection of light. Thus, acuity measurements of all kinds can give misleading impressions of the sensory tasks in which the nervous system is routinely engaged.

Minimum Separable Acuity and Minimum Angle of Resolution

When two dots or short line segments are made to approach each other in the visual field, a separation is reached at which the subject reports the presence of only one object. The critical angular spacing of the stimuli when they are just resolved is called the minimum angle of resolution (MAR) (Figure 9.1), a measure analogous to the two-point discrimination

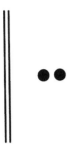

Figure 9.1. Examples of stimuli used to determine the MAR.

threshold in somatic sensation. The MAR is affected by many factors, including the brightness of the stimuli, the state of retinal adaptation, and the position of the stimuli on the retina. Humans usually can distinguish two stimuli separated by 30 seconds (30″) or 0.5 minute (0.5′) of arc when these are viewed with the fovea under optimal conditions of lighting and adaptation. This separation corresponds to about 2.5 μm on the retina, which is the spacing between adjacent foveal cones. This correlation led to the belief that two points can no longer be resolved when their images fall on adjacent cones; there must be at least one cone between the two images. As we shall see, the situation is more complicated than this.

Acuity of the MAR type is formally defined as the reciprocal of a spatial-discrimination threshold when the latter is expressed in minutes of arc. Thus, a MAR of 0.5′ would be equivalent to a minimum separable acuity of 2. In common usage, however, acuity is often expressed as the threshold itself.

Snellen Acuity

Practical measurement of visual acuity in humans is usually done with eye charts, of which the most common is that devised by Snellen (Figure 9.2). The Snellen chart uses letters of different sizes, which the subject is asked to identify. To distinguish an O from a C, an observer must be able to resolve a critical feature, namely the gap on the right side of the C. Most people can make this distinction when the gap subtends 1′ of arc. In principle, one could produce a Snellen chart with one line of letters, each letter printed with a critical feature that would subtend 1′ when the chart was exactly 20 feet from the observer. People with normal vision would be able to read the chart when it was 20 feet away. If the chart had to be closer than this, the observer's vision would be poorer than normal.

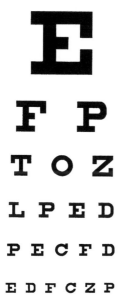

Figure 9.2. A Snellen chart.

In practice, Snellen charts contain several lines of letters, each line corresponding to a particular distance from the observer at which the critical features subtend 1′. The observer is placed a fixed distance from the chart, let us say 20 feet. At this distance, the line marked 20 on the chart is composed of letters with 1′ critical features. If the subject can read this line, but not the next smallest, he or she has 20/20 vision. The line marked 40 has letters whose critical features subtend 1′ at a distance of 40 feet. If the smallest letters that the subject can read are on the 40-foot line, it means that the subject must stand 20 feet from the chart to read a line that should be legible from 40 feet away. This subject has 20/40 vision, which is obviously worse than 20/20 vision. It is not unusual for some people to have 20/15 vision. Tests such as that using the Snellen chart reveal the best performance of the tested eye, which is normally that mediated by the fovea.

Charts using letters of the Roman alphabet provide a valid measure of acuity only for those familiar with this alphabet. Other charts employ devices such as Landoldt Cs, which are circles with gaps at different positions, and the subject is required to state whether the gap is up, down, right, or left. Visual acuity in infants can be assessed by measurement of visually evoked potentials or by tasks in which the infant's direction of gaze is attracted by bright patterns with elements of specified size. It is assumed that the infant's gaze will be attracted only by a pattern that he or she can resolve. The visual acuity of experimental animals can also be estimated by appropriate behavioral and electrophysiologic methods.

Grating Acuity

A grating is composed of alternating dark and light bars that can be presented at different levels of fineness and contrast and at different orientations. The period of a grating is the width of one complete cycle of dark and light regions, and its fineness is expressed in terms of its spatial frequency, the number of complete cycles of dark and light areas per degree of visual angle. Spatial frequency has its most precise meaning when applied to a grating whose luminance varies continuously and sinusoidally (Figure 9.3). Sinusoidal gratings lend themselves to the characterization of visual capacity in terms of Fourier theory.

Luminance is a physical measure related to the psychological perception of brightness. The luminance dimension of a grating is called its contrast and can be expressed quantitatively in different ways. A common convention is to define it as the maximum luminance difference between dark and light areas divided by the sum of these luminances:

$$(L_{hi} - L_{lo})/(L_{hi} + L_{lo})$$

where L_{hi} is highest and L_{lo} is lowest luminance. According to this formula, a black/white grating would have a contrast of 1 (or 100%), because L_{lo} would be zero.

Because the visual system detects some spatial frequencies better than others, grating acuity is usually summarized by plotting the reciprocal of threshold contrast for different spatial frequencies (Figure 9.4). The resulting curve is called the contrast sensitivity function (CSF) of the subject, which can be a human, a laboratory animal, or a single neuron in the visual system. When little contrast is needed, the CSF has high values, but goes to zero when the system is no longer able to distinguish a grating from a gray background of the same luminance as the average of the bright and dark areas of the grating (the space-average luminance). The range of spatial frequencies to which a system will respond is called the bandpass of the system. As shown in Figure 9.4, the bandpass of the human visual system contains higher frequencies than does that of the cat, which means that humans can resolve finer spatial detail than cats.

Grating acuity can be estimated roughly from the MAR, and vice versa, because a grating is simply repeated pairs of dark areas separated by light areas. Consider a square-wave grating in which the edges of the black bars

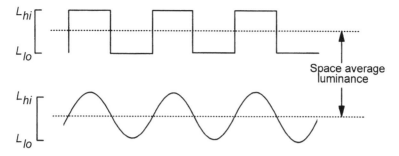

Figure 9.3. Luminance profiles of a square-wave grating (top) and a sinusoidal grating (bottom). An intensity level midway between the peaks and troughs of the grating is the space-average luminance (dashed line). L_{hi}, maximum luminance; L_{lo}, minimum luminance.

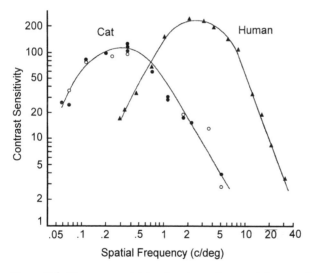

Figure 9.4. Contrast sensitivity functions of cat and human. Open and closed circles are data from two cats trained to press a lever at the appearance of a grating of variable contrast. Human data are from one observer. (Reprinted from S. Bisti and L. Maffei: Behavioral contrast sensitivity of the cat in various visual meridians. *Journal of Physiology* 241:201–10, 1974, with permission of The Physiological Society.)

are sharp. One could measure the MAR by extracting from this grating two black bars separated by a white bar. The MAR would be the smallest resolvable angle subtended by the white bar as the widths of the bars were decreased. If this turned out to be 0.5′ of arc, then one cycle of the grating would subtend 1′, and there would be 60 full sets of dark and light bars in the grating that could just be distinguished from a gray background of the same average luminance. It is of some interest that the CSF of humans falls to zero between 50 and 60 cycles per degree, as one might predict from a MAR of 0.5′ (Figure 9.4).

Vernier Acuity

Vernier acuity tasks assess the ability of the visual system to encode the relative positions of objects in the visual field. Examples of vernier acuity tasks are shown in Figure 9.5. In the example using two lines, the subject is asked to signal the smallest detectable lateral displacement of one line from the other. Displacements of a few seconds of arc can be detected in this task, and because this represents a retinal distance much smaller than the width of a foveal cone, vernier acuity is sometimes referred to as a hyperacuity. It should be noted, however, that this task is very different from that used in determining the MAR. In the vernier task, the brain is asked to make a decision about the relative positions of two or more extended objects that are clearly resolved. To accomplish this, the brain presumably can compare the macroscopic distribution of neural activity caused by the stimuli to some expected pattern that would occur were the stimuli perfectly aligned. The visual system is exquisitely sensitive to misalignments of this sort, as illustrated by the ease with which one notices the slightest tilt of a picture frame on the wall.

Physical Limits on Spatial Acuity

The spatial resolving power of a visual system depends on the quality of the retinal image and on the ability of the retina to transmit details in the image to the brain. Several physical factors affecting the quality of the retinal image were discussed in Chapter 3, including aberrations, refractive errors, diffraction at the edge of the iris, and scatter of light within the eye. These account for the fact that a bright point in object space is imaged as a blur circle on the retina. In attempting to separate physical factors from neural factors limiting spatial resolution, it is important to have a more quantitative measure of the performance of the optical system alone.

The modulation transfer function (MTF) of an optical system is analogous to the CSF. Whereas the CSF measures the frequency response of

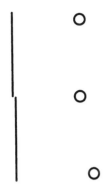

Figure 9.5. Examples of stimuli used in tests of vernier acuity. The subject is asked to detect the break in the line segment or the misalignment of the vertically distributed circles. The threshold is the visual subtense of the just-detectable horizontal displacement of the line segment or the misaligned circle.

the entire system (e.g., optics, retina, and brain), the MTF assesses only the frequency response of the optics. To determine the MTF, sinusoidal gratings of known contrast are presented in object space, and the contrast in the image is measured. The ratio of image contrast to object contrast as a function of spatial frequency is the MTF. Perfect transmission would give a value of unity, and no transmission a value of zero. In any real optical system there is always some reduction of contrast due to imperfections in the media, scatter, diffraction at apertures, and so forth. These factors affect some frequencies more than others. The MTF is usually described for objects like gratings whose contrast varies in only one dimension. It can, however, be extended to two dimensions.

The point-spread function is the two-dimensional distribution of light in the image of a point object, and it describes the potential blurring of every point in an extended object. It can be thought of as the quantitative equivalent of the blur circle. In a linear optical system, the image is simply the sum of the point spreads for every point in the object, with all the point spreads preserving the relative positions of their corresponding object points. The Fourier transform of the point-spread function is the two-dimensional modulation transfer function. The line-spread function, the distribution of light in the image of a line, is a one-dimensional version of the point-spread function (Figure 9.6). It is sometimes more convenient to determine the line-spread function than the point-spread function of a system.

The finite widths of the point-spread and line-spread functions of the human eye (Figure 9.6) indicate that no point in the visual field is imaged

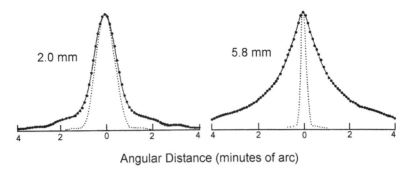

Angular Distance (minutes of arc)

Figure 9.6. Line-spread functions for the human eye at two pupil diameters. Note that the smaller pupil gives the narrower spread. The dotted line represents the diffraction image. These data were obtained from a living eye by analyzing the light reflected back out of the eye from the image of a bright line. (Reprinted from R. W. Campbell and R. W. Gubisch: Optical quality of the human eye. *Journal of Physiology* 186:558–78, 1966, with permission of The Physiological Society.)

as a perfect point on the retina. For two closely spaced point or line stimuli, the task of the detection system is to tell whether or not there are two peaks or, in other words, whether or not there is a trough in the distribution of light in the image. The ability to detect the trough will depend on a number of things, including the sampling area of the detectors and their spacing. This brings us to the subject of the limits set on resolution by the retina and central nervous system.

Retinal Determinants of Spatial Acuity

The fact that visual acuity is better in photopic vision than in scotopic vision shows clearly that retinal factors play major roles in spatial resolution. Also, visual acuity is much higher in the fovea than elsewhere, even though image quality does not vary greatly as a function of retinal position. Several specializations of the primate fovea contribute to its capacity to resolve fine detail, and many of these are also found in the foveas of other animals.

The retina is very thin at the fovea because the cells of the inner retina are displaced to the side (Figure 9.7). This permits light to reach the photoreceptors without passing through many structures that otherwise might degrade the image by scattering light. The absence of retinal vessels from the fovea also reduces the chance for light to be scattered by the vessels and the elements they contain (see Figure 2.2). This avascularity

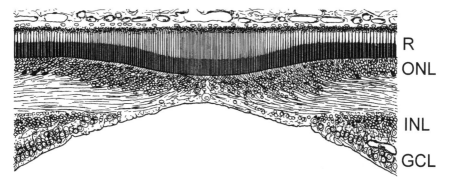

R
ONL
INL
GCL

Figure 9.7. Diagrammatic representation of the central fovea of the human retina. R, receptor layer; ONL, outer nuclear layer; INL, inner nuclear layer; GCL, ganglion cell layer. (Adapted from S. Polyak: *The Vertebrate Visual System*. Copyright 1957, The University of Chicago Press.)

does not impair the flow of oxygen and nutrients to the foveal photoreceptors, because these are supplied by the choroid.

The central fovea is occupied exclusively by cones (Figure 6.12), which are very thin and packed closely together. Thus, the cones sample the retinal image with a very fine grain. In the fovea the cones become rod-like in appearance, and their inner segments act like tiny light pipes, guiding incoming light to the outer segment (Figure 9.8). The thinness of the foveal cones also enhances resolution by limiting the effective light rays to those traveling almost parallel to their optic axes. Light that hits a cone at a steep angle passes out of it and is absorbed by the pigment epithelium (Figure 9.8). The effect is essentially to give each cone its own little pupil that selects those rays least affected by spherical aberrations. A reflection of this feature of the cones is seen in the Stiles-Crawford effect. When a narrow beam of light is directed through the pupil at the fovea, the effectiveness of the beam in evoking a visual response varies with the angle it makes with the visual axis.

There are no short-wavelength cones in the primate fovea (see Chapter 11), and a collection of yellow pigment in front of the fovea, the macula lutea, filters out short wavelengths. This reduces the effects of chromatic aberration due to stronger refraction of short wavelengths than of long wavelengths.

Each foveal cone is thought to contact one on-center and one off-center midget bipolar cell, and each midget bipolar cell in turn contacts a single midget ganglion cell that sends its axon into the optic nerve. Thus, the midget bipolar and ganglion cells provide single cones with a direct line

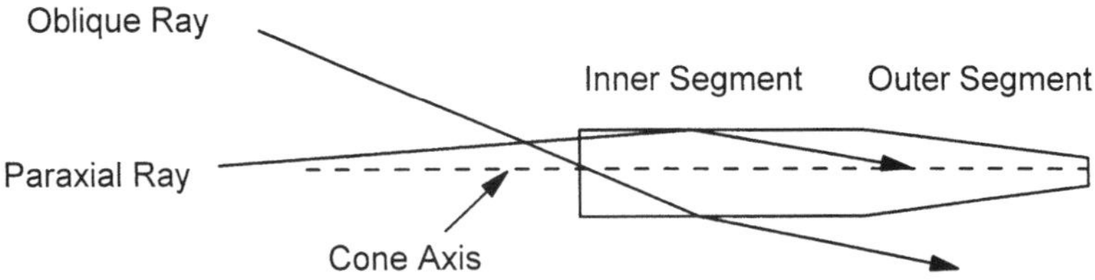

Figure 9.8. Schematic illustration of limited angle of acceptance of a cone. The paraxial ray undergoes internal reflection in the inner segment and reaches the photopigment in the outer segment. The oblique ray is refracted out of the cone to be absorbed in the pigment epithelium or choroid.

to the brain. The high densities of receptors, bipolar cells, and ganglion cells in the fovea translate into high magnification factors for the foveal representation centrally. Thus, the central neural representations of neighboring retinal points are farther apart when the points are in the fovea than when they are in the retinal periphery. Visual acuity and other spatial discrimination capacities are highly correlated with magnification factors in the visual pathway, as will be discussed later.

Does the Cone Mosaic of the Fovea Determine Maximum Acuity?

As mentioned at the beginning of this chapter, the separation of foveal cones (about 2.5 μm or 0.5') suggests that the CSF of humans should have a high-frequency cutoff at about 60 cycles per degree. The observed agreement between prediction and measurement is indeed highly suggestive. However, if one arranges to circumvent the degradative effects of the eye's optics on the retinal image, it can be demonstrated that the human retina can detect much higher spatial frequencies. This is accomplished by splitting a laser beam and directing the two secondary beams into the eye so that interference between them produces a sinusoidal grating where they combine at the retina. The separation of peaks and troughs can be varied by changing the relative positions of the two interfering beams. Gratings of very high spatial frequency created in this way are not perceived as regular alternating dark and light bands, but rather as patterns of curved, shimmering lines resembling moiré patterns, which the observer can distinguish from a uniform field of the same average brightness. Whereas subjects can detect the presence of structure in the retinal image, they cannot always identify the image as that of a grating of a particular orientation or spatial frequency. This distinction between detection and identification is critical here.

That the foveal cone mosaic theoretically might be able to detect a grating of very high frequency is illustrated in Figure 9.9. The circles represent the apertures of the individual cones formed by their inner segments. The cones are spaced 0.5′ apart, and the square-wave grating superimposed on them has a spatial frequency of 180 cycles per degree, far above the normal cutoff of the CSF. Yet cone B clearly receives more light than cone A, so their output signals should be different. If the brain can detect this difference, it can distinguish this grating from a uniform field of the same average intensity. Thus, there seems to be no reason why the foveal mosaic cannot detect spatial frequencies higher than 60 cycles per degree. Why does it not do this ordinarily?

The answer to this question requires a brief consideration of sampling theory. Consider the array of minute photodetectors spaced x degrees apart in Figure 9.10. The spacing, x, between the cells is called the sampling interval, and $1/x$ is the sampling frequency. The three sine waves represent the distributions of light in sinusoidal gratings of equal amplitude presented one after the other to the photodetectors, and the dotted lines indicate the points at which the sinusoids are sampled. Grating B is sampled twice in each cycle, grating A many times, and grating C only once in every few cycles. Observe that the outputs of the photodetectors will be different for gratings A and B, but identical for gratings B and C. In other words, any observer knowing only these outputs would not be able to tell grating C from grating B. No grating of lower frequency than B would give exactly the same output pattern as that grating. Therefore, grating B can be distinguished from all gratings of lower frequency, but not from some gratings of higher frequency (e.g., grating C).

The phenomenon in which a sampling array confuses higher frequencies with lower frequencies is called aliasing, because the higher frequencies look like the lower frequencies (i.e., they produce identical outputs from the sampling array). The sampling theorem states that the highest frequency that can be identified unambiguously is one that is sampled twice in each cycle of the waveform. Thus, if x in Figure 9.10 equals 0.5′ or 1/120 degree of arc, then all gratings of 60 cycles per degree or lower will be sampled at least twice in each cycle, and no two of them will yield exactly the same sample values and thus be confused with each other. The frequency $1/2x$, 60 cycles per degree in this case, is called the Nyquist frequency of the sampling array. If higher frequencies are present in the signal, they may produce exactly the same sample values as some lower frequencies and thus may not be distinguishable from these. Under such conditions, the output of the system is ambiguous because of aliasing.

Why, then, is aliasing not present during normal viewing? An excellent way to prevent aliasing is to limit a system's bandpass to frequencies below

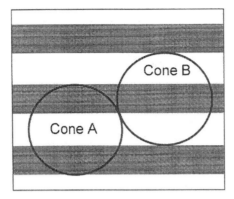

Figure 9.9. Interaction of a square-wave grating of 180 cycles per degree with two cones spaced 0.5' arc apart. Cone B receives more light than cone A.

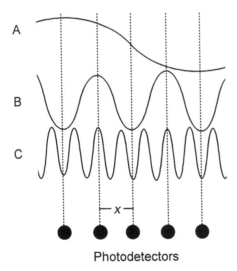

Photodetectors

Figure 9.10. Schematic illustration of aliasing. The light levels detected by the array of photocells are identical for gratings B and C, so C is aliased as B. Grating A is unambiguously encoded because no higher frequency can produce exactly the same pattern of outputs from the photocell array. x, the sampling interval.

its Nyquist frequency. In other words, design the system to screen out those frequencies that might be aliased. This appears to be the strategy adopted by the visual system. The combined effects of pupil size, aberrations, and all the other factors that degrade the retinal image effectively eliminate high spatial frequencies that the photoreceptor mosaic would mistake for lower frequencies. Moreover, cones sample the illumination of a small area, rather than a point on the retina, and this reduces their capacity to respond to high spatial frequencies in the image. Thus, the MTF of the eye's optics is closely matched to the bandpass and sampling interval of the foveal cones, as if the optics were designed to be as good as the retina and no better (or vice versa).

Retinal Magnification

A factor of obvious significance in determining visual acuity is the size of the retinal area devoted to a given region of visual space. This relationship is set by the posterior nodal distance and varies in different animals. A line subtending 1° of visual angle forms an image 290 μm long on the retina in the eye of an adult human. Thus, the linear retinal magnification of the human eye is about 290 μm per degree. This compares with retinal magnifications in macaque monkey and cat of about 223 and 207 μm per degree, respectively. If the foveas of two eyes have comparable cone densities (number per square millimeter), the eye with the larger retinal magnification has an effectively finer "grain" and should exhibit a higher spatial acuity.

Retinal Ganglion Cell Distribution and Visual Acuity

Although spatial resolution in the fovea appears to be set by the spacing between cones, this correlation does not hold for more peripheral regions of the retina. F. W. Weymouth first noted that human visual acuity declined with eccentricity at about the same rate as the distance between neighboring retinal ganglion cells increased. Subsequent studies in many species have attempted to quantify this relationship between acuity and the spatial density of the ganglion cells. The issue is complicated by the fact that retinas contain more than one class of ganglion cells, and within each class there may be on-center and off-center cells. If each class or subclass is considered to sample the retinal image independently, then each class has its own characteristic bandpass, sampling interval, and Nyquist frequency. As an example, the spatial distributions of X cells and Y cells in the cat's retina differ significantly, as do the bandpass properties of their receptive fields. It appears that the sampling properties of the β-cell array best match the visual acuity of the cat, but there is some disagreement whether the on-center and off-center cells need to be viewed as one sampling array or as two sampling arrays. A similar issue exists for P cells of the monkey's retina.

Spatial Resolution in Compound Eyes

The acuity of the invertebrate compound eye is also determined by optical and sampling factors. Spatial resolution is limited by the interommatidial angle, which depends on, among other things, the radius of curvature of the faceted cornea (Figure 9.11). In principle, the smaller this angle, the higher the sampling "grain" of the eye. Decreasing the diameters of the ommatidia allows the interommatidial angle to decrease, but it also increases the degree to which diffraction degrades the optical image, and a diminished quantal catch reduces the probability that faint signals will be detected. Many insects deal with this by varying the radius of curvature and ommatidial diameter in different regions of the eye (Figure 9.12). Those parts with the highest spatial resolution are relatively flat, so that interommatidial angles can be small, and they have large facets to reduce the optical problems inherent in narrow apertures. Thus, the region of the eye that appears as if it would have the coarsest sampling grain is actually the region with the best resolution.

Cortical Magnification and Visual Acuity

The feature of cortical organization that is most closely linked to visual acuity is the varying magnification of the visual field in the cortical retinotopic map. As has been noted, the foveal representation is much larger than that of any peripheral retinal area of equivalent dimensions. In fact, the magnification falls off continuously with distance from the fovea. The MAR, as one measure of visual acuity, also changes with distance from the fovea, but this angle increases as the cortical magnification factor decreases. The findings in a number of studies suggest that if the MAR is plotted graphically in the coordinate system of the cortical retinotopic map, this equivalent cortical distance is about the same everywhere in the visual cortex. This finding suggests that the neural machinery involved in determining the MAR is the same size everywhere in the cortex, and as a corollary, the MAR changes in the visual field because the mapping from retina to cortex is distorted.

This relationship was not revealed by actually replotting the MAR on the cortical map, but derives from the discovery that the cortical magnification factor, M, varies inversely with the MAR as a function of retinal eccentricity. The linear magnification factor describes the distance across the cortical map corresponding to a line subtending 1° in visual space. If the MAR at an eccentricity of 20° is 8° and the local cortical M is 0.7 mm per degree, the product MAR $\times$ M is 0.56 mm. This is the distance

Interommatidial Angle

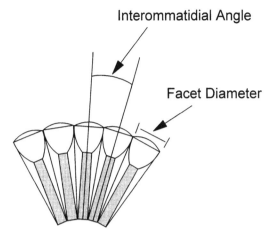

Figure 9.11. Interommatidial angle and sampling interval of a compound eye. The axes of the ommatidia vary with the curvature of the eye, and the angle between the axes of neighboring ommatidia determines the sampling interval of the eye. The greater the curvature, the larger the sampling interval.

across the cortical retinotopic map corresponding to an 8° line located 20° from the fovea.

Table 9.1 shows what happens when MAR measurements at several eccentricities are multiplied by the corresponding magnification factors. The effect is impressive. Whereas the MAR varies by a factor of 13.3 between 2.5° and 50°, the product of MAR and M is relatively constant. Similar translation-invariant equivalent cortical distances are found for grating acuity. Other psychophysical tasks, such as vernier acuity and minimal recognizable letter sizes, also yield relatively invariant cortical distances when multiplied by M, but the distances are not the same as those for the MAR. This suggests that different recognition or detection tasks engage cortical regions of different sizes during their execution.

Point Images in the Visual Pathway

The equivalent cortical distance obtained by multiplying M and MAR or any other limiting value of a spatial discrimination can be only an approximation to the amount of cortex involved, because any stimulus point lies in the receptive fields of cells distributed over a finite area of cortex. Thus, two point stimuli used to determine the MAR create two distributions of neural activity, and it is reasonable to assume that discrimination becomes impossible when the overlap of the two distributions exceeds

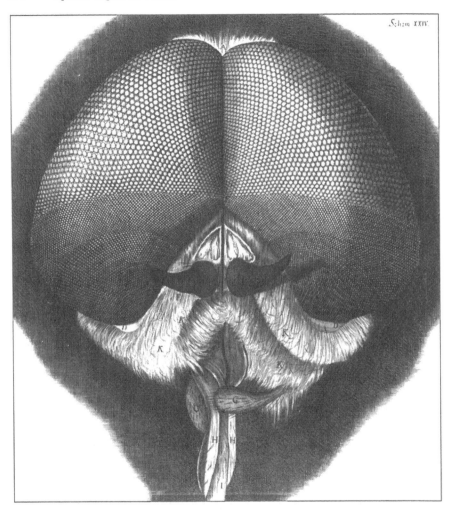

Figure 9.12. Drawing of a fly's eye showing variation in ommatidial size over the compound eye. The region of highest spatial resolution is at the top. (Reprinted from R. Hooke: *Micrographia*, 1665. Courtesy of the John Hay Library, Lownes History of Science Collection, Brown University.)

some critical value. A major task of visual neuroscience is to develop measures of the actual distributions of neural activity representing any visual stimulus, so that a complete account of the information about the stimulus available to the brain can be obtained.

A start in this direction is to determine the locations of all cells whose receptive fields contain a given visual point, a region that has been called

Table 9.1. *MAR scaled by cortical magnification factor M*[a]

Parameter	Eccentricity						
	2.5°	5°	10°	20°	30°	40°	50°
M (mm/deg)	3.87	2.35	1.31	0.70	0.48	0.36	0.29
MAR (deg)	0.018	0.028	0.044	0.080	0.116	0.163	0.210
MAR × M (mm)	0.070	0.066	0.058	0.056	0.056	0.059	0.061

[a]Values of M are from A. Cowey and E. T. Rolls: Human cortical magnification factor and its relation to visual acuity. *Experimental Brain Research* 21:447–54, 1974, as plotted in D. H. Foster, J. Thorson, J. T. McIlwain, and M. Biederman-Thorson: The fine-grain movement illusion: a perceptual probe of neuronal connectivity in the human visual system. *Vision Research* 21:1123–8, 1981. Values of MAR are from T. Wertheim: Ueber die indirekte Sehschärfe. *Zeitschrift für Psychologie* 7:172–87, 1984.

the neural point image. These are the only cells that "see" the point, so any cell that responds to a stimulus at that visual point must lie in the point image. This idea is easiest to understand if we first consider the point image among retinal ganglion cells, because the cells and their receptive fields are located in the same place. In general, the receptive fields are centered on the cell bodies, and for purposes of this discussion we ignore the center–surround organization and assume that the receptive fields are perfectly circular.

Given the assumptions just made, all points inside a ganglion cell's receptive field are no farther from the cell body than the radius of the receptive field. This means that the cells whose receptive fields just touch the point lie on a circle centered on the point, a circle whose radius is equal to that of a receptive field. Cells inside this circle (black cells in Figure 9.13) lie in the point image. Thus, the point image has the same size and shape as the receptive fields themselves. In this idealized situation, there is a perfect geometric reciprocity between receptive field and point image. If local receptive fields differ in size, the cells with the largest receptive fields can lie farthest from the point and still "see" it. Thus, the size and shape of the point image are set by the cells with the largest receptive fields.

The notion of point image is related to, but not identical with, the notion of coverage factor (i.e., the number of ganglion cells whose dendritic fields or receptive-field centers overlap at a given point) (see Chapter 6). The difference is obvious when one considers that the dendritic-field diameter and the spatial density of ganglion cells often tend to vary inversely. Thus the retinal coverage factor, which is given by the product of these

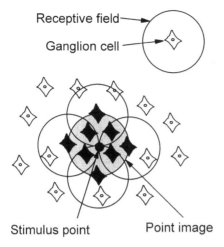

Figure 9.13. Geometry of point images in the retina.

two variables, can, in principle, remain constant while the point image varies in size.

Consider now the situation in a central structure, such as the striate cortex, that receives a retinotopic projection of the visual world. Here arises the major problem that the cells are in one place, the cortex, and the receptive fields have been plotted in retinal coordinates. We cannot repeat the process used in the retina, where cells and receptive fields are located in the same coordinate system. What we require is a relationship between points on the retina, where the receptive fields are known, and points in the cortex, where the cells actually live. This relationship is provided by a retinotopic map that accurately reflects the retinal origins of signals arriving at a given cortical point.

The first step in locating the boundaries of the cortical point image is to transfer the receptive-field boundaries from the coordinate system of the retina to that of the cortical map. This procedure in a sense "images" the receptive field into the new coordinate system, so the resulting profile has been called the receptive-field image (RFI) (Figure 9.14). Each point inside the RFI corresponds to a point inside the receptive field. A retinal point on the boundary of the receptive field has a corresponding point at the edge of the RFI.

Now, two other conditions will restore the situation that we have in the retina: (1) The cell bodies of the cortical neurons lie at some fixed point in the RFI. (2) The largest RFIs change little in size and shape over short distances. For simplicity, let us assume that the cell bodies lie at the

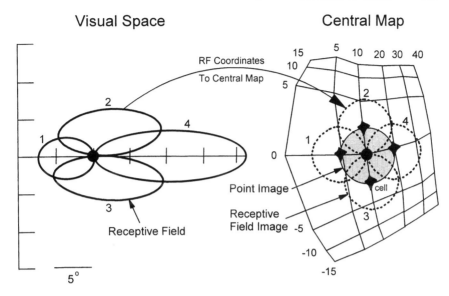

Figure 9.14. Receptive-field images and point images in a central map. The receptive-field images are obtained simply by transferring the boundary coordinates of the receptive fields to the coordinate system of the retinotopic map.

center of perfectly circular RFIs that do not vary in size or shape over a small region of the cortical map. Here, then, is the geometric situation of the idealized retina of Figure 9.13, except that now a cortical cell can lie no farther from a map point than the radius of its RFI and still see the point (Figure 9.14). Any point outside its RFI will correspond to a retinal point outside its receptive field. Once again, the cells with the largest RFIs can lie farthest from a map point and still have the corresponding retinal point inside their receptive fields. Thus, the cells with the largest RFIs lie at the edge of the cortical point image. By the same logic that holds in the retina, the point image will be identical in size and shape to the largest RFIs of the cortical cells, and if the assumptions listed earlier are made, its size can be estimated by multiplying the diameter of the largest receptive fields recorded at a site by the local cortical magnification factor. The same principles apply, but the analysis becomes more complex, as the simplifying assumptions are relaxed.

In general, the assumptions made here are approximately correct for the striate cortex. One exception is that neighboring cells sometimes have receptive fields that do not perfectly overlap in visual space. This is called receptive-field scatter and can be interpreted to mean that the cell bodies are not located at identical places in their RFIs. It is necessary to incorporate this scatter into any calculations of point-image size if the scatter is large relative to the size of the RFIs. There are several ways to do this, depending on the assumptions one makes about the nature of the scatter. The main result, though, is that the boundaries of the point image are not sharp, but probabilistic. For instance, one might define the edge of the point image as that place where no more than 1% of the cells see the point.

Estimates of point-image size in the monkey's striate cortex indicate that it decreases from the foveal area to the representation of the periphery. Point-image diameter may reach 10 mm in the foveal representation, but is about 1 mm in peripheral parts of the map. Neighboring visual points obviously have overlapping point images, so this analytic machinery is shared by nearby points. It is also clear that the foveal point image contains many hypercolumns (see Chapter 8), because these are only about $1-2$ mm in diameter. Thus, the analytic superiority of foveal vision over peripheral vision may reflect not only the large magnification factor the fovea enjoys in striate cortex but also the fact that any stimulus point viewed by the fovea is analyzed by a much larger number of cells than points imaged on the peripheral retina.

Up to now we have spoken as though there were only one point image in the striate cortex. This is useful as a way of introducing the subject, but it may be important to assess the point image in each of the functional subsystems of the cortex, because these differ in their afferent and efferent connections and in the geometry of their receptive fields. For instance, the cells in layer 4 have small receptive fields, and the two eyes remain relatively separate in the map, which implies that here there exist two small point images for a given point in the visual field. This fact may be important for stereoscopic vision or spatial acuity, whereas the large size of the single point image of layer 5 may ultimately be related to the control of gaze through the cortico-tectal projection arising from this layer.

Further Reading

Cowey, A., and Rolls, E. T. (1974). Human cortical magnification factor and its relation to visual acuity. *Experimental Brain Research* 21:447–54.

Dow, B. M., Vautin, R. G., and Bauer, R. (1985). The mapping of visual space onto foveal striate cortex in the macaque monkey. *Journal of Neuroscience* 5: 890–903.

Goldsmith, T. H. (1990). Optimization, constraint, and history in the evolution of eyes. *Quarterly Review of Biology* 65:281–322.

Grinvald, A., Lieke, E. E., Frostig, R. D., and Hildisheim, R. (1994). Cortical point-spread function and long-range interactions revealed by real-time optical imaging of macaque monkey primary visual cortex. *Journal of Neuroscience* 14:2545–68.

Hubel, D. H., and Wiesel, T. N. (1977). Ferrier lecture: Functional architecture of macaque monkey visual cortex. *Proceedings of the Royal Society of London* 198: 1–59.

Levi, D. M., Klein, S. P., and Aitsebaomo, A.P. (1985). Vernier acuity, crowding and cortical magnification. *Vision Research* 25:963–77.

McIlwain, J. T. (1988). Point images in the visual system: new interest in an old idea. *Trends in Neurosciences* 9:354–8.

Polyak, S. (1957). *The Vertebrate Visual System.* University of Chicago Press.

Rowe, M. H. (1991). The functional organization of the retina. In *Vision and Visual Dysfunction. Vol. 3: Neuroanatomy of the Visual Pathways and Their Development,* ed. B. Dreher and S. R. Robinson, pp. 1–68. Boca Raton: CRC Press.

Van Essen, D. C., Newsome, W. T., and Maunsell, J. H. R. (1984). The visual field representation in striate cortex of the macaque monkey: asymmetries, anisotropies and individual variability. *Vision Research* 24:429–48.

Wehner, R. (1981). Spatial vision in arthropods. In *Handbook of Sensory Physiology. Invertebrate Visual Centers,* vol. 7, part 6C, ed. H. Autrum, pp. 287–616. Berlin: Springer-Verlag.

Weymouth, F. W. (1958). Visual sensory units and the minimal angle of resolution. *American Journal of Ophthalmology* 46:102–13.

Williams, D. R. (1985). Aliasing in human foveal vision. *Vision Research* 25:195–205.

CHAPTER 10

BINOCULAR VISION AND DEPTH PERCEPTION

When the eyes face the front, the central part of the visual field is imaged on both retinas (see Figure 4.4). This bestows certain advantages for depth perception, but also creates a formidable problem for the brain: how to ensure that the two retinal images are transformed to yield a unified perception of the part of the visual field seen by both eyes. Failure to achieve this, which sometimes happens in pathological conditions of the nervous system, results in diplopia, the perception that there are two objects when there really is only one. Diplopia can be demonstrated by pushing gently on the skin at the side of one eye to misalign the two visual axes.

Binocular Single Vision

The encoding of the two retinal images of a single object to yield a unique perception results in perceptual fusion of the two images. In discussing fusion, it is important to distinguish between it and two other phenomena, fixation and focus. If the visual axis of one eye is directed at an object so that the image is positioned on the fovea, the eye is said to fixate the object. It is possible to deliberately place an image outside the fovea, but the term "fixation" is generally used to mean foveal fixation. The fixated object will be in focus only if its distance from the eye and the power of the eye's optics permit the formation of a crisp retinal image. The common expression "he focused on such and such" confounds the two very different concepts of fixation and focus and even implies that fusion has occurred and attention is directed to the object. By positioning the images of an object on appropriate points in the two retinas, not necessarily on the foveas, a single or fused perception of the object can be obtained. Fusion does not require that the object be fixated or that its images be in focus, but it does require that the object be viewed binocularly.

If one monocular image of an object is located at a particular point in, say, the left eye, fusion is possible as long as the other monocular image is positioned somewhere within a small region around the retinotopically corresponding point in the right eye, a region called Panum's fusional area. The retinotopic correspondence between the fused images need not be exact, hence the term "fusional area" instead of "fusional point." Because this relationship applies to either eye, the fusional mechanism links small regions of the retinas, not just points. The external manifestation of the linkage of fusional areas in the two eyes is that an object appears single when it is located within a slab-shaped volume of visual space, and double when it is located outside this volume. Empirical determinations of this region of visual space, called Panum's zone of single vision, have shown that it contains the fixation point and bends around the subject, growing wider in the periphery (Figure 10.1).

Of particular interest with respect to the mechanisms underlying fusion is evidence that the boundaries of Panum's zone are not fixed, but depend to some degree on the kind of stimuli used and on the history of such stimulation. For instance, the zone widens as the spatial frequencies in the test stimuli decrease. Also, certain fusional phenomena exhibit a kind of hysteresis; once fusion has been achieved, the retinal images can be moved to what would ordinarily be diplopic conditions without interrupting fusion. It is as if the fusional mechanism can "lock on" to a pattern and, within limits, adjust the boundaries of Panum's zone to prevent loss of fusion. These observations suggest that fusion is not simply a process linking fixed zones in the two retinas but rather one that exhibits significant dynamic characteristics.

There exists at present no adequate neurophysiologic theory of how the brain actually achieves perceptual fusion of the two retinal images. It seems certain that the anatomic projection of the retinal inputs to a single cortical area makes a fundamental contribution to this process, but important questions remain. Does some particular spatial congruity between the neural representations of the two images have to occur in the primary visual cortex before fusion is possible? What neural mechanisms are responsible for linking Panum's fusional areas in the two eyes and for providing the dynamic properties of this linkage? Answers to these questions await further research.

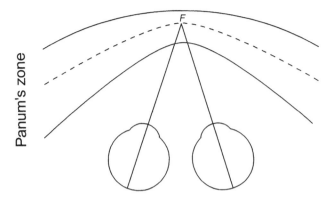

Figure 10.1. Schematic view of Panum's zone of single vision. Objects located between the solid curved lines are seen as single; objects outside this region appear double. A line through the center of Panum's zone has been proposed as the locus of visual points that are imaged on functionally corresponding retinal points. *F*, fixation point.

Depth Vision and Stereopsis

A human observer uses monocular and binocular cues to assess distances to objects in the external world. Monocular cues are perhaps the most important in daily life and are more than adequate for most of the tasks we perform. People who have only one functional eye drive automobiles successfully, although they must be concerned with a diminished field of view.

The important monocular cues to distance are size, occlusion, perspective, and motion parallax. The known sizes of familiar objects, such as a person or a house, provide an immediate indication of how far away they are from the observer. Also, if one object partially occludes a person's view of another, the first object is closer than the second. Parallel lines, such as the edges of a road or the intersections of walls and ceiling, appear to converge, and the relative distance between objects can be estimated by their positions along these converging trajectories. "Motion parallax" refers to the fact that nearby objects appear to move more than distant objects when the viewer's position changes. Thus, when one is riding in a car, the telephone poles beside the road appear to pass by much faster than do trees located several hundred feet away.

The many monocular cues to depth in a visual scene are perhaps why closing one eye does not make the scene appear flat or two-dimensional. Nonetheless, when viewing objects with both eyes, most people experience a vivid sense of depth not present with monocular viewing. This phenomenon, known as stereopsis, is not the same as fusion and should not be confused with it. There are individuals who cannot make stereoscopic discriminations, but nonetheless have normal fusion. Objects lying just outside Panum's zone of single vision cannot be fused, but they still evoke a perception of stereoscopic depth and appropriate vergence movements of the eyes.

Stereoscopic vision depends on the fact that the two eyes are separated horizontally and consequently have slightly different views of objects located different distances away. In Figure 10.2, the two eyes fixate the point F, which is imaged on the foveas. It is evident that rays from the dot through the nodal points form different angles, α and β, with the visual axes of the two eyes, so the images of the dot lie at different distances from the two foveas. Said another way, the retinal coordinates of the two images are not the same in the two eyes. The difference between these coordinates is the retinal disparity in the images of the dot. Retinal disparity can have horizontal and vertical components. The images of multiple external objects have differing absolute disparities with respect to the fovea and different relative disparities with respect to each other.

The visual system can detect retinal disparities as small as 2″ of arc, which is a much higher resolution than the MAR and qualifies stereoacuity as a so-called hyperacuity. The actual values obtained in tests of stereoacuity depend on a number of factors, such as type of stimulus, number of disparity cues, duration of exposure, eccentricity, and fixation distance.

Crossed and Uncrossed Disparities

The relative positions of the two retinal images of an object viewed binocularly provide a critical clue to whether the object is nearer or farther than the fixation point. In Figure 10.3, the two eyes fixate a point, F, on a transparent screen. When object A, located behind the screen, is viewed with the right eye alone, it appears to be farther to the right of F than when it is viewed with the left eye. This can be seen by extending a line from each eye's nodal point to A. Where the lines intersect the screen, A_r lies to the right of A_l. In this case, the retinal images of A are said to have uncrossed disparity because the monocular visual images have the same relative positions as the two eyes. In contrast, point B lies between the observer and the screen, and lines through B and the nodal points reverse the relative positions of B_r and B_l. In this case, the right eye sees B to the left of where it is seen by the left eye. Thus, the images of B are said to have crossed disparity.

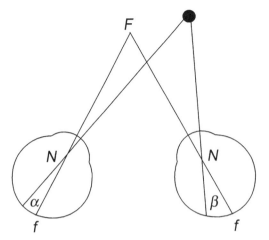

Figure 10.2. Geometry of binocular disparity. The two eyes fixate point *F*. The dot is imaged on loci with disparate retinal coordinates, illustrated by the difference between angles α and β. The disparity is horizontal in the diagram but may also have a vertical component. *N*, nodal point; *f*, fovea.

The meanings of crossed and uncrossed disparities can be appreciated directly in the following way. Position one index finger about 6 inches from the nose in the midline and the other at arm's length. Fixating the near finger, adjust the position of the far finger so that its double image is centered on the fixation point. Closing the left eye causes the left image of the far finger to disappear, and closing the right eye causes the right image to disappear. Now fixate the far finger and center the double image of the near finger on the fixation point. Closing either eye causes the image on the opposite or crossed side to disappear. In this case the disparity associated with the near object causes its perceived monocular directions to appear crossed. In a word, objects between the observer and the fixation point have images with crossed disparity; objects beyond the fixation point have images with uncrossed disparity.

Corresponding Points and Horopters

In discussing Panum's fusional areas it was noted that a pair of such areas would have similar retinotopic coordinates. Research on binocular vision and stereopsis has been concerned to discover if a more precise linkage between retinal coordinates can be identified, one that actually ties a point

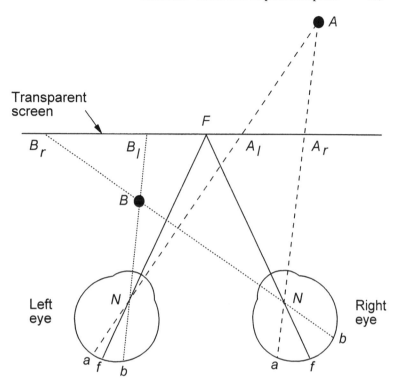

Figure 10.3. Crossed and uncrossed disparities. Disparity of A is uncrossed; disparity of B is crossed. F, fixation point; f, fovea; a and b, retinal images of A and B; N, nodal points. A_r, A_l, B_r, B_l, apparent positions of A and B relative to F when viewed monocularly.

in one retina to a point in the other. Such a linkage would associate what are called <u>corresponding points</u>, but because this term can refer to a number of substantially different concepts, it must be used with care. Its connotations fall into two general classes: <u>Geometrically corresponding points</u>, as the name implies, are defined by geometry alone; <u>functionally corresponding points</u> are defined by various perceptual tasks involving the two eyes. The lines or surfaces formed by visual points imaged on corresponding retinal points, whether defined geometrically or functionally, are sometimes called <u>horopters</u>, from Greek *horos* (boundary or limit) and *opter* (observer). "Horopter" is a problematic term because it has more than one meaning. There are as many horopters as there are ways of defining corresponding points.

Geometrically Corresponding Retinal Points: The Vieth-Müller Circle

In foveate animals, such as primates, geometrically corresponding points are defined as retinal loci that have exactly the same retinotopic coordinates in the two eyes or, said another way, lie the same distance and direction from the fovea. If one imagines that the two retinas are removed and one is placed against the other in the same orientation and with the foveas in perfect alignment, a pin driven through both retinas would pass through geometrically corresponding points. In the plane defined by the two convergent visual axes there exists a locus, the Vieth-Müller (V-M) circle, that passes through the fixation point and the nodal points of both eyes (Figure 10.4A). The V-M circle has the property that points on its circumference are imaged at geometrically corresponding points on the two retinas. This follows from the geometric rule that triangles inscribed in a circle and sharing a side have equal angles opposite that side (for proof, see Figure 10.4B and its legend). This principle requires that $\angle FNQ$ and $\angle FN'Q$ in Figure 10.4A be equal, because they share the side FQ (dotted in Figure 10.4A). Consequently, their opposites, $\angle fNq$ and $\angle f'N'q'$, are also equal. Points q and q' therefore occupy geometrically corresponding points.

Theoretically, a vertical geometric horopter lies in the mid-sagittal plane where all points have zero azimuth and identical elevations for each eye. It is evident, though, that many lines in that plane share this property, so no unique geometric locus exists. However, a unique functional locus can be identified, as will be discussed later.

Empirical or Functional Determinations of Retinal Correspondence

Empirical studies of retinal correspondence are based on the assumption that properly chosen perceptual tasks requiring the use of both eyes will reveal how points in one retina are linked to points in the other. Unhappily, the hope of finding a unique linkage has been frustrated largely by the fact that different perceptual tasks lead to different configurations of corresponding points.

One traditional approach defines corresponding retinal points as those that represent the same monocular visual direction from the observer. To identify these, a subject fixates a point straight ahead and views a vertical rod positioned at various distances to one side of the fixation point (Figure 10.5). Observing the rod through an apparatus that allows one eye to see the top half and the other to see the bottom half of the rod, the subject moves the rod back and forth until the top and bottom halves appear to

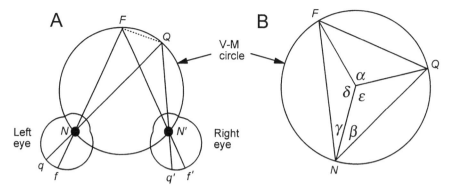

Figure 10.4. (A) The V-M circle passes through the fixation point, F, and the two nodal points N and N'. Q, any point on the V-M circle; f, fovea; q and q', retinal images of Q. (B) Construction for proof that triangles inscribed in a circle and sharing a side have equal angles opposite that side. N, F and Q are the same as in Figure 10.4A; angles α, δ, and ε are formed by radii of the circle, and the triangles containing them are therefore isosceles. $\angle FNQ = \beta + \gamma$; $\delta = 180° - 2\gamma$; $\varepsilon = 180° - 2\beta$, so $\alpha = 360° - (\delta + \varepsilon) = 360° - (180° - 2\beta) - (180° - 2\gamma) = 2(\beta + \gamma) = 2\angle FNQ$. Thus, the inscribed angle at point N is always half as large as α, the vertex angle of a triangle based on the same chord but located at the center of the circle. Because α remains constant regardless of the location of N, the angle at N will remain constant for any position of N on the circle, including N' in panel A. Thus, in panel A, $\angle FNQ = \angle FN'Q$, so opposite angles $\angle fNQ$ and $\angle f'N'Q'$ must also be equal, and q and q' are the same distance from their respective foveas.

belong to a single object. The position of the rod is marked, and it is moved to another site in the visual field, and then the test is repeated. The points where the rod is seen as single correspond to locations on the two retinas that, when stimulated monocularly but simultaneously, represent the same egocentric direction from the observer. This approach yields the nonius horopter, which does not correspond in space exactly to the V-M circle.

Other empirical approaches to locating corresponding retinal points require the subject to identify visual points that appear to lie in a frontal plane containing the fixation point or, alternatively, points that appear to lie the same distance from the subject. Not surprisingly, the resulting apparent frontoparallel plane and equidistant horizon differ from each other and from the nonius horopter and V-M circle. A fusional criterion assumes that points on a line down the middle of Panum's zone are imaged on corresponding retinal points. Other proposals define corresponding retinal points as the loci of maximal stereoacuity at a given fixation distance,

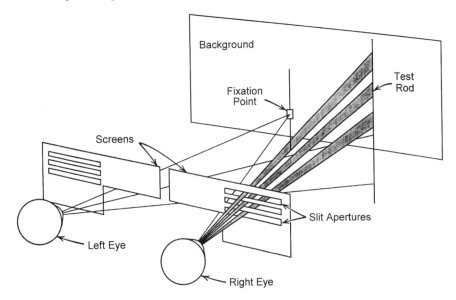

Figure 10.5. Method for obtaining the nonius horopter. The subject's right eye views the top of the target line through a slotted screen, while the left eye views the bottom of the target. The subject moves the target until the interrupted upper part of the target (which appears as a dashed line) is directly above the continuous lower part. At this point the separate images in the two eyes appear to arise from an object at one location in visual space whose image coordinates in the two eyes must therefore correspond to a unique direction from the viewer. (Adapted from K. N. Ogle: *Researches in Binocular Vision*, 1950. Philadelphia: W. B. Saunders Co., by permission of The Mayo Foundation.)

or the region in which the sudden appearance of stimuli elicits no fusional (convergent or divergent) eye movements.

Because different empirical methods identify different patterns of corresponding retinal points and, accordingly, different horopters, neither of these concepts refers to a unique characteristic of the visual system. None the less, the various manifestations of retinal correspondence reflect properties of the mechanism underlying binocular vision and stereopsis and must be accounted for in any adequate theory of this mechanism.

Random-Dot Stereograms

A key task of the brain is to determine which features in the two retinal images represent single features in the external scene and, at the same

Figure 10.6. Example of a random-dot stereogram. When viewed in a stereoscope or when "free-fused" by fixating behind or in front of the page, a figure appears at a different depth than the background. (Reprinted from B. Julesz: *Foundations of Cyclopean Perception*. The University of Chicago Press. Copyright 1971, Bell Telephone Laboratories.)

time, to ignore spurious matches when there are two or more identical features in the images. This constitutes what is called the correspondence problem. Scenes with many features that can be easily confused with one another often give rise to false correlations and ambiguous perceptions of depth. An example is when one is looking through a cyclone fence and is able to fuse the repeating pattern of the wires by fixating at a variety of points in the distance. Objects in a natural visual scene generally have distinguishable shapes, which can be used in the identification process, but this renders such scenes difficult to use in investigating how the brain solves the correspondence problem.

A considerable advance was made when it became possible experimentally to eliminate monocular cues but still provide disparity cues in visual stimuli. The basic technique uses a pair of monocular stimuli composed of apparently random distributions of small elements that reveal no shapes or objects when viewed alone (Figure 10.6). The patterns in these random-dot stereograms are identical, with one exception. A set of elements in one member of the stimulus pair (e.g., in a square area) is displaced horizontally by a small amount, so that these elements have a finite disparity with respect to their counterparts in the other member of the pair. When the two patterns are fused (e.g., by using a stereoscope), the disparate set of dots is seen as a shape floating in front of or behind a plane formed by the background elements. This kind of stimulus has been applied fruitfully in a wide range of psychological and physiologic studies by B. Julesz and others. For instance, many visual illusions persist when presented as random-dot stereograms, indicating that the mechanism responsible for the illusion is located at or above the point in the visual pathway where the inputs from the two eyes are combined. Some animals can be trained to respond to the depth cues encoded in random-dot stereograms, permitting physiologic observations on the stereoscopic mechanisms in the brain.

The study of random-dot stereograms has established an important distinction between two levels of stereoscopic processing. To fuse the two monocular halves of the stereogram, the subject must match the local features of one with those of the other, the process of local stereopsis. Because there are many possible spurious matches in a random-dot stereogram, there must be a higher-level process, global stereopsis, that recognizes the embedded figure and ratifies, as it were, a specific pattern of local matches. The mechanism responsible for global stereopsis is so powerful that a continuous edge can sometimes be perceived in parts of a figure where local disparity cues are not present. How local stereopsis and global stereopsis are implemented in the brain is a major research question.

Neural Basis of Fusion and Stereopsis

Fusion and stereopsis are subjective phenomena, so a full understanding of their neural basis requires an understanding of the mechanism of perception itself. One can say with some confidence that this remains shrouded in mystery. Neurophysiologic studies have documented the responses of single neurons in the visual pathway to binocular stimulation, and recent neural theories of fusion and stereopsis have been based largely on these findings. Here we shall discuss the most influential of these theories, namely, that single neurons of the visual cortex encode depth by responding to stimuli with restricted retinal disparities. Such neurons are viewed as labeled lines for disparity.

Most neurons of the striate cortex respond to stimulation of either eye, meaning that they have a receptive field on each retina. Furthermore, the most effective activation occurs when a stimulus is imaged on both retinal receptive fields at the same time. The stimuli themselves are in the outside world, so it is useful to think of the projection of the retinal receptive fields into visual space. Imagine that the receptive fields of a cortical neuron are luminous spots on the retina that are projected by the optics of the eye like searchlight beams into visual space (Figure 10.7). A stimulus object located anywhere along the beam from either eye will be "seen" by the cortical cell, because the image will lie in the retinal receptive field of that eye. If the beams from the two monocular receptive fields intersect

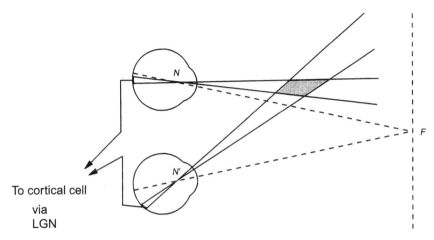

Figure 10.7. Receptive-field disparity and optimal stimulus position. In this diagram, the monocular receptive fields of a cortical cell are superimposed in front of the fixation plane containing the fixation point F. An object located in the shaded area is imaged on both monocular receptive fields of this cell. Such a cell is optimally stimulated by near objects whose retinal images have crossed disparity. N, N', nodal points.

at some distance from the subject (hatched area in Figure 10.7), a stimulus located at this intersection will lie simultaneously in both of the cortical cell's receptive fields. At this point, the binocular receptive fields are said to be superimposed or to coincide in visual space, and studies of binocular cortical neurons indicate that many respond best, and some only, when a stimulus lies just at that point of superposition.

Because the region of receptive-field superposition in the diagram of Figure 10.7 lies between the eyes and the fixation point, the receptive fields themselves must occupy retinal loci that are not in geometric correspondence, just as do the images of point B in Figure 10.2. In other words, this cortical cell exhibits receptive-field disparity and in consequence responds preferentially to stimuli a certain distance away. Moving the stimulus toward or away from the point of receptive-field superposition decreases its effectiveness and may even inhibit the cell.

Research in both cats and monkeys has shown that different cortical cells have binocular receptive fields that are superimposed at different distances from the animal. In other words, the population of cells exhibits a range of receptive-field disparities or, what is the same thing, a range of preferred stimulus distances. In the cat, most cells respond best to stimuli located on an approximately semicircular line, concave toward the subject, that passes through the fixation point. Other cells respond best to stimuli in front of or behind this line, forming a slab of space that is wider in the periphery than near the fixation point. The similarity of this distribution to the shape of Panum's zone is noteworthy (cf. Figure 10.1). Certain cortical cells of the macaque are tuned for stimuli producing images with crossed, zero, and uncrossed disparity, and some of these appear to prefer a very narrow range of disparities (Figure 10.8). Other cells respond preferentially to near or far stimuli, but are not as narrowly tuned as those of Figure 10.8.

If it is assumed that these cells signal the disparity of stimuli to which they are responding, then the brain could perhaps use their discharge to estimate relative distances in the visual scene. Definitive support for this hypothesis has yet to emerge from experimental studies, but certain observations are consistent with it. For instance, rearing conditions that reduce the binocularity of cortical neurons also reduce an animal's capacity to respond to cues encoded in random-dot stereograms. However, the fact that many disparity-tuned cells respond vigorously to monocular stimulation poses a problem for the idea that such cells are labeled lines for distance or depth. Their responses to monocular stimulation would imply disparity when there was none. Also, the discharge of disparity-tuned cells varies with other stimulus parameters, such as direction of motion (Figure 10.8), so a given rate of discharge does not uniquely represent a particular disparity in the retinal images.

There is evidence from electrophysiologic recordings in monkeys that the preferred disparities of striate cortical neurons may change dynamically under certain conditions. B. C. Motter and G. F. Poggio recorded eye position in alert macaques while monitoring the locations of the receptive fields of binocular cortical neurons and observed that the receptive fields remained relatively stationary on the tangent screen despite movements of the eyes. This means that the receptive fields of these neurons were moving on the retinas in such a way that their projected directions in visual space remained relatively constant. It is as if the discharge of the cortical cell were "tuned" to a particular direction in visual space rather than to a single disparity value in its retinal connections. The mechanism responsible for such dynamic disparity tuning is not known, but one possibility is that the return projection from striate cortex to the LGN is part of a circuit that can effect small spatial adjustments in the convergent inputs from monocular geniculate laminae to binocular cortical neurons.

Stereopsis and Fusion in the Mid-sagittal Plane

Stimuli immediately in front of or behind the fixation point are imaged, respectively, on both temporal retinas or both nasal retinas (Figure 10.9).

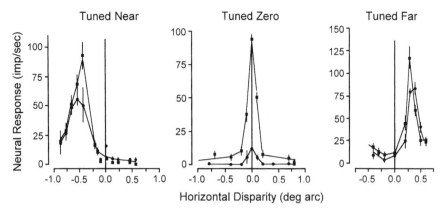

Figure 10.8. Examples of disparity tuning curves from striate cortical neurons of the alert macaque. To produce such curves, the responses of a single neuron are recorded while images of varying disparity are projected on the retinas. These cells are tuned for crossed (left), zero (center), and uncrossed (right) disparities. The two curves in each panel represent responses of the same cell to opposite directions of stimulus motion. (Adapted from G. F. Poggio, R. Gonzalez, and F. Krause: Stereoscopic mechanisms in monkey visual cortex: binocular correlation and disparity selectivity. *Journal of Neuroscience* 8:4531–50, 1988, with permission of the Society for Neuroscience.)

This means that the two monocular signals representing one such stimulus are sent to opposite hemispheres. One possible route for uniting the monocular neural representations of such a stimulus is the corpus callosum, which connects the parts of areas 17 and 18 representing the vertical midline of visual space. D. Mitchell and C. Blakemore found that patients with transection of the corpus callosum were unable to state whether objects presented in the vertical midline were nearer or farther away than the fixation point, although these patients had no difficulty making such discriminations in the right or left visual hemifields.

The Vertical Horopter

Binocular vision in the mid-sagittal plane has received far less attention than vision on the horizon. As noted earlier, however, points on the mid-sagittal plane have zero azimuth and identical elevations in the two eyes, so one would expect there to be a locus in this plane analogous to certain of the horizontal horopters. Helmholtz argued that the locus of points perceived singly in this plane is a line through the fixation point that is tilted away from the observer at the top and passes through the floor near

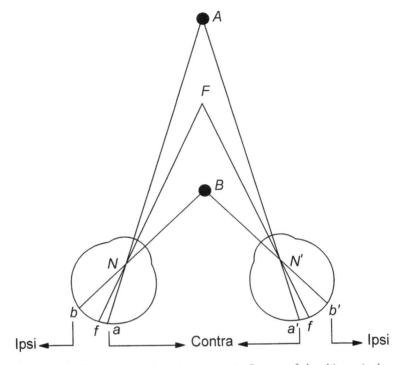

Figure 10.9. The problem of midline stereopsis. Because of the chiasmatic de-
cussation, signals representing the left and right retinal images of midline objects
A or B are sent to separate hemispheres, precluding any direct binocular convergence of the geniculo-cortical afferents onto single cortical neurons.

the observer's feet. His argument was based on psychophysical observations
suggesting that the retinal meridians linked by the fusional mechanism to
represent points in the mid-sagittal plane are not truly vertical and parallel, but rather are rotated away from each other at the top.

The likely anatomic correlates of these linked meridians are the nasotemporal raphés of the two eyes (i.e., the lines passing through the foveas
that separate ganglion cells projecting to ipsilateral and contralateral cerebral hemispheres). It is not known if the nasotemporal raphés of humans
are, in fact, rotated away from each other at the top, but we shall assume
that they are to illustrate how this would affect the geometry of retinal
correspondence. Observe that visual points imaged on the raphé of one eye
must lie in a plane formed by lines from the raphé through the nodal
point of the eye (Figure 10.10A). When both eyes are used, the intersection of these planes is the locus of points that are imaged simultaneously

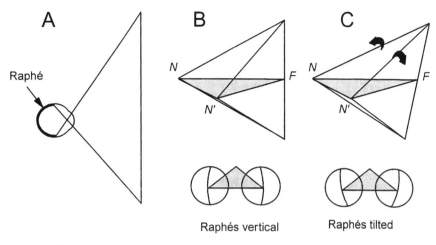

Figure 10.10. The vertical horopter. (A) Side view of the eye. Projection of the nasotemporal raphé through nodal point into visual space forms a plane. Any point on that plane is imaged on the raphé. (B) The intersection of raphé projection planes from two eyes is vertical if the raphés are vertical. (C) Intersection of raphé projection planes tilts away at the top when raphés are tilted away from each other superiorly. Shaded area is the fixation plane containing the nodal points N and N' and the fixation point F.

on the raphés of the two eyes. If the raphés were vertical, the intersection of the planes would be a line normal to the fixation plane defined by the intersecting visual axes (Figure 10.10B). However, because the raphés and their associated projection planes are (presumably) rotated away from each other superiorly, the intersection is a line tilted away from the observer at its top (Figure 10.10C). Thus, object points below the fixation plane will be imaged on corresponding retinal points only if they lie between the observer and the fixation point, whereas object points above the fixation plane must lie beyond the fixation point to be imaged on the raphés.

Using the nonius criterion (Figure 10.5), K. Nakayama and colleagues confirmed this tilt in the locus of midline points representing a common visual direction. Also, physiologic studies of binocular cortical neurons by M. Cooper and J. D. Pettigrew in both cat and owl showed that the receptive fields of such neurons tended to have crossed disparity when located below the fixation point, and uncrossed disparity when located above it. Thus, stimuli that optimally activated such cells would have to be located on a line in the mid-sagittal plane that was tilted away from the animal at its top. Should these cells be encoding stereoscopic depth information, the findings suggest that depth perception is optimized si-

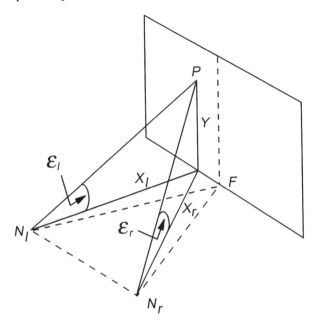

Figure 10.11. Absence of geometric correspondence for points in the visual quadrants.

multaneously near the animal's feet and at the point of fixation, an arrangement with obvious advantages for visually guided behavior.

Stereopsis and Fusion in the Visual Quadrants

As noted earlier, unless visual points are located on the V-M circle or in the mid-sagittal plane, their images will fall on geometrically noncorresponding retinal points. Points in the quadrants of the visual field satisfy neither of these conditions and in fact are always imaged on geometrically noncorresponding retinal points. Why this is so is illustrated in Figure 10.11. Because point P is farther from the right eye than the left, the angle ε_r must be smaller than angle ε_l if the two rays from the nodal points are to intersect at P. Thus, point P is imaged on retinal loci having different elevations and, consequently, a vertical disparity. These loci will also have a horizontal disparity unless P is located on a cylindrical surface perpendicular to the fixation plane through the V-M circle.

Many cortical cells have receptive fields at noncorresponding retinal points, so one might think that this takes care of points in the visual quadrants. Observe, however, that the rays from the nodal points to P

intersect only because angles ε_r and ε_l are uniquely matched to the distances X_l and X_r to yield the same value of Y at the screen. If the viewing distance changes, but angles ε_r and ε_l remain constant, these same two rays do not intersect anywhere in visual space. One always passes over the other. If we now think of the two rays as analogous to the beams from a cortical cell's receptive fields, as in Figure 10.7, these fields are perfectly superimposed at only one fixation distance. Thus, a cortical cell that responds optimally to a stimulus at P, because this is where the centers of its receptive fields coincide, can have its capacity to respond reduced if the fixation distance changes. A similar difficulty for retinal correspondence arises when fixation is not symmetric, but is to one side or the other of the straight ahead.

One way around this difficulty would be to adjust the disparity tuning of cortical cells dynamically, as reported by Motter and Poggio in the study described earlier. Such a mechanism could vary the preferred disparity of cortical neurons to maintain adequate responsiveness of cortical cells under changing viewing conditions. Dynamic disparity tuning would have implications for the neurophysiologic theory of depth perception described earlier, which assumes that certain cortical cells represent labeled lines for disparity or depth. If the preferred disparity of a cortical cell changes with viewing conditions, the neuron's discharge becomes ambiguous with regard to depth unless fixation distance and angle are incorporated in the encoding process.

Further Reading

Barlow, H. B., Blakemore, C., and Pettigrew, J. D. (1967). The neural mechanism of binocular depth discrimination. *Journal of Physiology* 193:327–42.

Bishop, P. O. (1987). Binocular vision. In *Adler's Physiology of the Eye*, 8th ed., ed. R. A. Moses and W. M. Hart, Jr., pp. 619–89. St. Louis: Mosby.

Cooper, M. L., and Pettigrew, J. D. (1979). A neurophysiological determination of the vertical horopter in the cat and owl. *Journal of Comparative Neurology* 184:1–26.

Helmholtz, H. (1924). *Treatise on Physiological Optics*, vol. 3, ed. J. P. C. Southall. New York: Dover.

Julesz, B. (1971). *Foundations of Cyclopean Perception*. University of Chicago Press.

Mitchell, D. E., and Blakemore, C. (1970). Binocular depth perception and the corpus callosum. *Vision Research* 10:49–54.

Motter, B. C., and Poggio, G. F. (1990). Dynamic stabilization of receptive fields of cortical neurons (VI) during fixation of gaze in the macaque. *Experimental Brain Research* 83:37–43.

Nakayama, K., Tyler, C. W., and Appleman, J. (1977). A new angle on the vertical horopter. In *Abstracts of the Association for Research in Vision and Ophthalmology, Annual Meeting*, p. 82.

Ogle, K. N. (1950). *Researches in Binocular Vision.* Philadelphia: Saunders.

Ogle, K. N. (1962). The optical space sense. In *The Eye*, vol. 4, part 2, ed. H. Davson, pp. 211–417. New York: Academic Press.

Regan, D., Frisby, J. P., Poggio, G. F., Schor, C. M., and Tyler, C. W. (1990). The perception of stereodepth and stereomotion: cortical mechanisms. In *Visual Perception. The Neurophysiological Foundations*, ed. L. Spillman and J. S. Werner, pp. 317–47. New York: Academic Press.

Richards, W. (1967). Apparent modifiability of receptive fields during accommodation and convergence and a model for size constancy. *Neuropsychologia* 5: 63–72.

Shipley, T., and Rawlings, S. C. (1970). The nonius horopter. I. History and theory. *Vision Research* 10:1225–62.

Tyler, C. W. (1991). The horopter and binocular fusion. In *Vision and Visual Dysfunction. Vol. 9: Binocular Vision*, ed. D. Regan, pp. 19–37. Boca Raton: CRC Press.

CHAPTER 11

COLOR VISION

One of the main tasks of vision is to distinguish objects from their backgrounds, which at a minimum requires detection of spatial differences in patterns of retinal illumination. This capability is greatly enhanced if the organism can also discern differences in the wavelengths of the light forming the retinal image. These spectral or chromatic patterns can also be useful in the identification, as well as the detection, of important objects such as food sources or predators. The spectral composition of the retinal image of a given object depends on the spectral content of the incident light, the object's reflectance characteristics, and to some extent the differential absorption of certain wavelengths in the ocular media before light reaches the retinal photoreceptors. It is the photoreceptors that first dissect the retinal image into its chromatic components, and in the vertebrate retina this process depends on the cones.

Color vision generally requires the presence in the retina of two or more photopigments with different spectral sensitivities. As described previously, the photopigments of all animals are composed of an opsin, a large, membrane-spanning protein, and the chromophore, 11-*cis* retinaldehyde. When the chromophore absorbs a light quantum, it changes shape and activates the opsin, which then functions as a catalyst for further reactions in the photoreceptor (see Chapter 5). Retinaldehyde by itself is colorless, but when combined with the opsin its geometry is modified, and the combination becomes a photopigment that absorbs light in the visible range. Changes in one amino acid group at critical points in the opsin can significantly alter the spectral sensitivity of the opsin-chromophore combination. Because the amino acid sequence of the opsin is determined genetically, mutations throughout evolution have produced a wide range of photopigments with spectral sensitivities often matched to the ecological niches of the animals employing them.

The Trichromatic Theory of Color Vision

Modern theories of color vision began with Sir Isaac Newton, who knew that white light could be split by a prism into a spectrum of colored components and that combining some of these could recreate the sensation of white. He postulated that vibrations of different magnitude in the "ether" resulted in the perception of color when they excited comparable vibrations in the ends of the optic nerves. Building on this idea, Thomas Young surmised that different colors are perceived when different "vibrations" of the light interact with special "particles" in the retina. He reasoned that not every point on the retina could contain all the particles required to capture every vibration, so there must be a small number of broadly tuned particles with overlapping sensitivities, each vibration affecting the particles in different ratios. White light appears white because it excites all of the particles about equally. He then argued that there must be at least three different kinds of particles. If there were but one, it would not be able to tell the difference between changes in the amplitude of a vibration and changes in the frequency of the vibration. If there were only two, there should be one particular vibration that would excite the two particles equally and look like white light. Young did not see a white region in the spectrum produced by a prism, so he concluded that there must be at least three particles. This theory was later elaborated by Helmholtz and expounded in what is generally known as the Young-Helmholtz trichromatic theory of color vision. It has been confirmed in its essentials by modern methods, which show that there are normally three types of cones in the human retina, and each type contains a different pigment. The spectral sensitivity of the cone is essentially determined by the absorption spectrum of its photopigment.

Young's notion that a single, broadly tuned particle could not provide unambiguous information about the wavelength of light has more recently been called the principle of univariance. This principle says simply that a photoreceptor can only increase or decrease its output, so its signal is ambiguous as to whether the change is due to a shift in the wavelength or to a change in the intensity of the incident light. The photoreceptor of Figure 11.1A contains a pigment that captures light of wavelengths λ_1

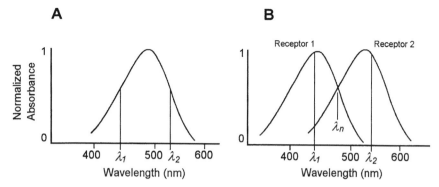

Figure 11.1. Wavelength discrimination by photoreceptors. The curves represent the relative capacities of the pigments to absorb light of different wavelengths, which essentially determines the spectral sensitivity of the photoreceptor. (A) The principle of univariance. A single receptor type can only signal more or less energy at some wavelength within its spectral sensitivity range. It responds identically to stimuli of wavelengths λ_1 and λ_2 if their intensities are equal. (B) In a two-pigment system, wavelengths λ_1 and λ_2 affect receptors 1 and 2 in different ratios, but there is one wavelength, λ_n, that appears white because it affects both receptor types equally.

and λ_2 equally well. If these lights are of equal intensity, the cell gives identical responses to both stimuli. Lights of other wavelengths can produce the same response if their intensities are suitably adjusted.

If there were two receptors with broad but overlapping tuning curves (Figure 11.1B), most wavelengths would affect the two receptors to different degrees, and no wavelength would give exactly the same ratio of activation as any other. By comparing the responses of the two receptors, the nervous system could distinguish virtually any wavelength from another. However, there would be two situations in which the receptors would be affected equally: when all wavelengths were present, as in white light, and when one wavelength fell at the intersection of the two spectral absorbance curves (λ_n in Figure 11.1B). This latter wavelength, called the neutral point, would be confused with white light. As noted earlier, Young did not detect this neutral point in himself and concluded that there must be at least three receptor mechanisms, as in fact there are in most people. Individuals who lack one of the cone pigments exhibit such a neutral point.

Trichromatic vision could work if there were three types of photoreceptors, each containing a different pigment or, alternatively, three types of photoreceptors, each containing three pigments in a ratio different from those of the other two types. This issue was settled definitively in the 1960s by investigators who used a technique called microspectro-photometry to measure the spectral absorbance of the pigments in single cones. It was shown that humans have three types of cone pigments, with peak absorbances at short, medium, and long wavelengths. Although these pigments are often called blue, green, and red, their peak absorptions do not coincide with wavelengths producing these hues, and it is preferable to refer to them as S, M, and L pigments. Their spectral absorption characteristics are illustrated in Figure 11.2. The letters S, M, and L are also used to designate the three types of cones.

It is evident that visible light of a given wavelength affects at least two and sometimes all three cones. Slight changes in wavelength result in slight changes in the ratio of activities among the cones. Although the output of any one cone is ambiguous with respect to the wavelength of the incident light, each wavelength is associated with a unique ratio of cone activities. This type of transformation results in an ensemble code, because the nature of the stimulus is encoded in the pattern of activity of a number of cells, rather than in the isolated activity of one cell.

The trichromatic nature of color vision explains certain effects of combining light of different wavelengths. For instance, by adding a red-appearing wavelength to one that appears green, and adjusting the intensities appropriately, one can produce the same ratio of S:M:L cone activity that results from presenting a single wavelength that appears yellow (Figure 11.2). Similarly, by combining blue and yellow lights of the proper intensity, one can affect all three cones equally, mimicking the effects and appearance of white light.

Trichromacy also explains why any colored light can be matched by some combination of no more than three other colored lights. A standard way of assessing color matches is to present the subject with a bipartite field (Figure 11.3), half of which contains the light to be matched, and the other half some mixture to be adjusted by the observer until the two half fields appear identical. As we shall see later, most people use virtually the same wavelength combinations in the same intensities to match a given color. Departures from "normal" trichromacy can be detected when individuals use combinations that differ from the normal pattern.

Because color vision has its greatest value for species that are active during the day, it is not surprising that wavelength discrimination is particularly well developed in animals such as birds, reptiles, and some fish whose evolution can be traced through long lines of diurnal ancestors. Hummingbirds, chickens, and pigeons may have as many as four (or more) different cone photopigments, allowing them to make fine discriminations over a wide part of the spectrum visible to humans and into the ultraviolet.

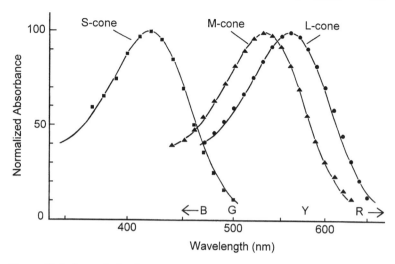

Figure 11.2. Spectral absorbances of human S-, M-, and L-cone pigments. B, G, Y, and R refer to the regions of the spectrum that appear to humans as blue, green, yellow, and red. (Adapted from H. J. A. Dartnall, J. K. Bowmaker, and J. D. Mollon: Microspectrophotometry of human photoreceptors. In *Color Vision*, ed. J. D. Mollon and L. T. Sharpe, pp. 69–80. London: Academic Press. Copyright 1983, with permission of Academic Press, Ltd.)

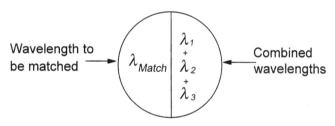

Figure 11.3. Diagrammatic representation of a bipartite field. The subject is required to match the hue in the left part of the field by combining different wavelengths in the right half of the field.

The cones of certain birds, turtles, and amphibians also contain colored oil droplets that may further refine their spectral selectivity. Acting as a filter, the oil droplet can limit the wavelengths that reach the photopigment in the cone outer segment (Figure 11.4). In principle, a color vision system could be constructed from cones containing one photopigment and one of several kinds of oil droplets, but vertebrate evolution does not seem to have adopted this strategy.

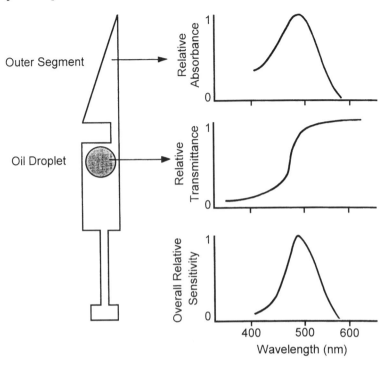

Figure 11.4. Effect of an oil droplet in the cone inner segment. Light must pass through the droplet to reach the outer segment. The droplet cuts off the shorter wavelengths and narrows the overall spectral sensitivity of the cone relative to that of its photopigment (compare the top and bottom panels on the right).

In invertebrates, as in vertebrates, wavelength discrimination is usually based on the presence of more than one pigment type in the photoreceptors. Insects have also developed other strategies for shaping the spectral sensitivities of their ommatidial photoreceptors. Alternating layers of material in the corneal facet can serve as interference filters, permitting a restricted range of wavelengths to reach the photopigment. Neighboring ommatidia can be tuned, as it were, to different parts of the spectrum by varying the filtering properties of the cornea. The photoreceptors of certain flies contain additional pigments that serve as "antennas," capturing photons of ultraviolet light and transmitting the energy to rhodopsin to initiate the visual process. Virtuosity in wavelength discrimination seems to have reached something of a peak in the mantis shrimp, which inhabits the shallow waters above coral reefs. In one part of its compound eye there are at least eight spectrally distinct types of photoreceptors. The eye achieves this by means of a variety of combinations of screening pigments and photopigments. Moreover, another part of the eye contains photoreceptors sensitive to the polarization angle of light.

Color Deficiencies

It has long been known that certain individuals fail to perceive color differences that are apparent to others. Although these individuals are said to be "color-blind," most of them can make wavelength discriminations, and it is more accurate to speak of their vision as being color-deficient. Truly color-deficient individuals are lacking one or more of the three cone photopigments. The prefixes prot- (= 1), deuter- (= 2), and trit- (= 3) are combined with -anopia to indicate the absence respectively of the long-, medium-, and short-wavelength photopigments. Thus, we have protanopia, deuteranopia, and tritanopia in individuals called protanopes, deuteranopes, and tritanopes. These individuals are dichromats, because their color vision is based on two, rather than three, wavelength-sensitive mechanisms. As predicted by Thomas Young, dichromats have neutral points; that is, they confuse particular spectral wavelengths with white. Dichromats also need lights of only two wavelengths to match any other color. Individuals lacking two or all three of the cone mechanisms cannot discriminate one wavelength from another, have no color vision, and are known as monochromats.

Some people with trichromatic vision, as determined by color-matching studies, do not use the same pattern of wavelengths as normals in their matches. These anomalous trichromats have three types of cones, but the spectral sensitivity of one of the pigments is shifted along the wavelength axis relative to its normal counterpart. Depending on which pigment is affected, these individuals are said to be protanomalous, deuteranomalous, or tritanomalous.

Studies of the spectral sensitivity of different areas of the human retina have revealed that the center of the fovea lacks the S-cone mechanism and is therefore tritanopic. Certain histologic stains that label S cones confirm that they are absent from the very center of the fovea. Adding to this foveal dichromacy is the macula lutea, a concentration of yellow screening pigments in front of the foveal area that reduces the amount of short-wavelength light reaching the foveal and parafoveal cones.

Tritanopia is rare, but protanopia and deuteranopia occur relatively frequently, and mostly in males. The typical pattern of inheritance of these latter two forms of dichromacy is sex-linked recessive and indicates that the defective genes are located on the X chromosome. Because the human female has two X chromosomes, each normally carrying the M and L pigment genes, the normal genes on one chromosome can compensate for missing or defective genes on the other. The pigment genes are not present on the Y chromosome, so a male who inherits an X chromosome defective in the M or L pigment gene will be a dichromat. Protanopia and deuteranopia provide excellent examples of the sex-linked recessive pattern of inheritance (Figure 11.5). In most families the condition skips generations, appearing in the grandsons of grandfathers who are themselves dichromats. These grandsons have inherited the defective X chromosome that their mothers received from the grandfather. A female must inherit defective X chromosomes from both her mother and her father to be a protanope or deuteranope.

Using the methods of molecular biology, J. Nathans and colleagues succeeded in locating the gene for the S pigment's protein on chromosome 7 in humans. A single gene for the L pigment and multiple copies of the M pigment gene were found on the X chromosome. The gene for rhodopsin was traced to chromosome 3. These investigators determined the DNA sequence of the pigment genes and assessed their degree of relationship from the deduced amino acid sequences of their protein products. All of the photopigments shared some degree of sequence similarity, suggesting that they had a common ancestor, but the L and M pigments showed a 96% mutual sequence identity (Figure 11.6), indicating that they evolved relatively recently, probably from duplication of a gene on the X chromosome. Nathans and colleagues also confirmed that protanopes and deuteranopes lack functioning genes for the L and M pigments, respectively. The corresponding anomalous trichromacies are associated with detectable modifications in these genes.

Most living primates with color vision are dichromats. This may reflect a long evolutionary period in which the ancestors of modern primates were active only at night. New World monkeys, such as the squirrel monkey, have a gene for a short-wavelength pigment but, unlike their Old World cousins, bear only a single photopigment gene on the X chromosome, a gene coding for one of three possible middle- to long-wavelength pigments. Many females of these species have two different longer-wavelength genes, one on each X chromosome, and thus have trichromatic vision. The males, with only one X chromosome and an S-cone pigment gene, are dichromats. Humans and Old World monkeys are trichromats, apparently having acquired an extra photopigment gene on the X chromosome by duplication and modification of the single ancestral gene located there. The genetic analysis of cone pigments has led to the proposal that the primate fovea and its associated midget bipolar and ganglion cells developed first to maximize spatial resolution. With the later emergence of two types of cone pigments, the fovea became dichromatic and capable of mak-

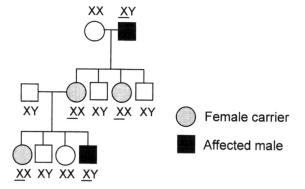

Figure 11.5. Pattern of inheritance that is sex-linked and recessive. The abnormal X chromosome is underlined. If this chromosome carries the gene for only one photopigment, the affected males are dichromats.

ing wavelength discriminations as well. Working together with the extra-foveal S cones, the "new" M and L cones bestowed trichromacy on the retinas of humans and Old World monkeys. Presumably, New World monkeys evolved in isolation from this process and developed a different pattern of cone specializations.

Opponent-Color Theory

The Young-Helmholtz trichromatic theory accounts for a number of phenomena encountered in color vision, but not for all. For instance, while the theory can predict that a properly adjusted combination of a long wavelength and a medium wavelength cannot be distinguished from a third wavelength we would call yellow, it does not explain why the combination *looks* yellow instead of greenish red or reddish green. Also, the color of a stimulus object depends on the colors surrounding it (simultaneous color contrast) and on the colors seen immediately before it (successive color contrast).

Insight into these phenomena has been provided by what is known as the opponent-color theory, introduced by E. Hering in 1878 and developed extensively by L. Hurvitch and D. Jameson. Hering postulated that vision is mediated by three visual processes, two chromatic and one achromatic. In one chromatic process, yellow and blue are paired in an opponent or antagonistic relationship. In the other, red and green form the opponent pair. Among other things, this theory accounts for the observation that one cannot see both members of an opponent chromatic pair at the same place at once. Thus, there are no reddish green, greenish red, bluish yellow,

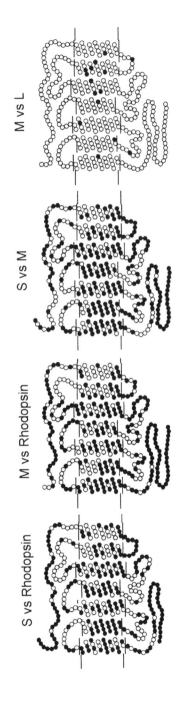

M vs L

S vs M

M vs Rhodopsin

S vs Rhodopsin

○ Same   ● Different

Figure 11.6. Protein similarities of the various visual pigments. Empty circles represent amino acids that are common to the two pigments being compared. S, M, and L indicate short-, medium-, and long-wavelength pigments, respectively. (Adapted from J. Nathans, D. Thomas, and D. S. Hogness: Molecular genetics of human color vision: the genes encoding blue, green and red pigments. *Science* 232:193–202. Copyright 1986, American Association for the Advancement of Science.)

or yellowish blue hues. The achromatic process mediates the perception of blackness and whiteness.

The fundamental postulates of Hering's theory have been borne out by observations on retinal ganglion cells of several species, including primates. In the latter, P cells are often excited by one color of the Hering pairs and inhibited by the other. Thus, a cell may be excited by a red light and inhibited by a green light, firing when the latter is turned off. This cell would be classified as having a red-on:green-off receptive field and would fail to respond to the combination of red and green light if the excitatory and inhibitory effects cancelled each other. Other cells have response types of green-on:red-off, blue-on:yellow-off, and yellow-on:blue-off, although off responses to blue lights are rare. The color-opponent receptive fields may have a center–surround organization as well, for instance, a red-on center and green-off surround. These response types are also found in the LGN and visual cortex, but in the latter one also finds so-called double-opponent cells. These cells may, for example, be red-on:green-off in one part of the receptive field and green-on:red-off in other parts. Double-opponent cells are found in the retina of the goldfish.

An obvious question for visual scientists is how the various cone inputs are combined at the ganglion cell to yield the signals sent forward to the brain. It is these signals that presumably determine the color perceptions evoked by the visual scene. Several models have been proposed, and the basic idea can be illustrated by the highly oversimplified scheme of Figure 11.7. Here we consider only the effects on ganglion cells and omit the mediating bipolar cells that must be involved. The red-on:green-off cell receives excitatory input from an L cone and inhibitory input from an M cone. A yellow-on:blue-off cell receives excitatory input from both M and L cones and inhibitory input from an S cone. The reciprocal organizations are also shown. Cells in the achromatic channel receive either excitatory or inhibitory input from all three cone types.

If one assumes that the discharge of each cell type evokes the perception shown under the arrows in Figure 11.7, one can see how the opponent mechanisms would give rise to certain phenomena not fully explained by the trichromatic theory. Consider the color-mixture phenomena described earlier:

Green + *red* = *yellow.* The opponency of M- and L-cone inputs to the red:green cells prevents them from firing, but because the combined M- and L-cone inputs excite the yellow-on:blue-off cell and inhibit the blue-on:yellow-off cell, the message sent to the brain says "yellow."

Blue + *yellow* = *white.* Light that appears yellow affects both M and L cones and disables the red:green cells that receive opponent input from

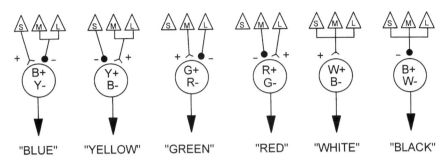

Figure 11.7. Hypothetical connections for constructing color-opponent receptive fields of retinal ganglion cells. The color named under each arrow indicates the perception assigned (hypothetically) to the discharge of that cell. The hyperpolarizing effect of light on the cones has been taken into account, so the plus and minus signs represent respectively the net excitatory and inhibitory effects of cone illumination. Among other things, this cartoon ignores the intervening bipolars, the estimated weightings of the various connections, and evidence for S-cone input to the "red" process that accounts for violet hues.

these cones. Blue light is detected by the S cones that are connected to the yellow:blue cells in opponent fashion. Thus, the combination of blue light and yellow light also inactivates the blue:yellow system because of the opponent nature of the S and M+L inputs. The "black" channel is also inhibited, leaving only the "white" system to respond.

If one is exposed to a bright color, say red, for a period of time and then looks at a gray or white background, one sees a green afterimage. This is an example of successive color contrast, which may also be explained by the opponent-color mechanisms. Prolonged viewing of the red stimulus (or exposure to a bright red flash) induces adaptation of the L cones, which become less sensitive than the M cones. Subsequent exposure to a white light, containing both medium and long wavelengths, has a greater effect on the M cones than on the L cones, and the "green" system is differentially activated. The same argument holds for the other opponent systems as well. Simultaneous color contrast requires the addition of lateral interactions between chromatic channels and may involve the double-opponent cells mentioned earlier, but this important phenomenon is still poorly understood.

Central Representation of Chromatic Information

The central mechanisms of color vision appear to involve parallel processing similar to that observed for other aspects of the retinal image. Thus, color-opponent cells of the primate retina project to the LGN but not to the midbrain, and as discussed in Chapter 7, the P retinal ganglion cells carrying chromatic information send their axons to the parvocellular layers, but not the magnocellular layers, of the LGN. Lesions of the parvocellular layers of the LGN eliminate wavelength discriminations in the affected part of the visual field, indicating that the P-cell pathway is essential to color vision.

Cells exhibiting color-opponent behavior are found throughout the striate cortex, but appear to be especially prevalent in the small regions that stain heavily for the mitochondrial enzyme cytochrome oxidase (see Figure 8.6). The color-opponent cells in these cytochrome oxidase blobs, as they are called, tend not to be orientation-selective. The blobs project preferentially to the regions of area 18 that do not stain positively for cytochrome oxidase, the so-called interstripes. There is little consensus on the parcellation of color-processing regions beyond this, but it is clear that more than one area or one circuit in the cerebral cortex is involved. For instance, a region of the occipito-temporal cortex known as area V4 (see Figure 8.14) appears to have a high concentration of color-sensitive cells, but removal of this area produces only a mild deficit in wavelength discrimination. Lesions of ventral occipito-temporal cortex in humans sometimes produce a selective loss or impairment of color vision, though recognition of shapes may be partially or completely preserved. This condition is called cerebral achromotopsia, and such patients perceive colors as faint and desaturated.

Color Constancy

The colors of natural objects remain relatively constant despite variations in the spectral content of the light reaching them. Thus, leaves appear green in the very different lights of early morning, high noon, and dusk. This phenomenon is called color constancy and is believed to result from high-level cerebral mechanisms that compare the chromatic signals arising from large areas of the retina to "correct" the color perception for variation in the ambient light. Color constancy has resisted explanation on the basis of photoreceptor or low-level opponent mechanisms.

Further Reading

Cronin, T. W., Marshall, N. J., and Land, M .F. (1994). The unique visual system of the mantis shrimp. *American Scientist* 82:356–65.

D'Zmura, M., and Lennie, P. (1986). Mechanisms of color constancy. *Journal of the Optical Society of America* A3:1662–72.

Goldsmith, T. (1990). Optimization, constraint and history in the evolution of eyes. *Quarterly Review of Biology* 65:281–322.

Hamdorf, K. (1979). The physiology of invertebrate visual pigments. In *Handbook of Sensory Physiology*, vol. 7, part 6A, ed. H. Autrum, pp. 145–224. Berlin: Springer-Verlag.

Hering, E. (1878). *Zur Lehre vom Lichtsinne.* Vienna: Gerolds Sohn.

Hsia, Y., and Graham, C. H. (1965). Color blindness. In *Vision and Visual Perception,* ed. C. H. Graham, pp. 395–413. New York: Wiley.

Hurvitch, L. M. (1981). *Color Vision.* Sunderland: Sinauer.

Jacobs, G. H. (1981). *Comparative Color Vision.* New York: Academic Press.

Jacobs, G. H. (1986). Color vision variations in non-human primates. *Trends in Neurosciences* 9:320–3.

Menzel, R. (1979). Spectral sensitivity and colour vision in invertebrates. In *Handbook of Sensory Physiology,* vol. 7, part 6A, ed. H. Autrum, pp. 501–80. Berlin: Springer-Verlag.

Mollon, J. D., and Sharpe, L. T. (eds.) (1983). *Colour Vision.* London: Academic Press.

Nathans, J. (1989). The genes for color vision. *Scientific American* 260:42–9.

Nicol, J. A. C. (1989). *The Eyes of Fishes.* Oxford: Clarendon Press.

Schiller, P. H. (1993). The effects of V4 and middle temporal (MT) area lesions on visual performance in the rhesus monkey. *Visual Neuroscience* 10:717–46.

Stavenga, D. G., and Schwemer, J. (1984). Visual pigments of invertebrates. In *Photoreception and Vision in Invertebrates*, ed. M. A. Ali, pp. 11–61. New York: Plenum.

Zeki, S. M. (1973). Colour coding in rhesus monkey prestriate cortex. *Brain Research* 53:422–7.

Zrenner, E., Abramov, A., Akita, M., Cowey, A., Livingstone, M., and Valberg, A. (1990). Color perception: retina to cortex. In *Visual Perception. The Neurophysiological Foundations,* ed. L. Spillmann and J. S. Werner, pp. 163–204. New York: Academic Press.

CHAPTER 12

OCULAR MOVEMENTS

Eyes admit light from a limited range of directions, so it is important that an animal be able to redirect its gaze to examine its surroundings. This is achieved by movements of the body, the head, and usually the eyes as well. Animals also use vision to guide movements of the body, and one would like to understand the way in which visual sensory information is transformed into motor commands. The relative simplicity of ocular movements, as compared, for instance, to movements of the arm, makes them useful for the study of such sensorimotor transformations.

The angle over which an animal can sweep its direction of gaze by moving its eyes alone is called its oculomotor range. This varies from species to species. The oculomotor range of a cat is about 50°, and that of macaque monkeys and humans about 90°. Owls rotate their tubular eyes only about 3° in the orbits, but a very mobile head compensates for this. Chameleons can rotate their turret-like eyes independently. Invertebrates employ a variety of mechanisms to explore their visual environments. Compound eyes that are fixed to the exoskeleton are moved by head or body movements. Jumping spiders are able to move their retinas behind the fixed lenses of their ocelli, and certain copepods also have mobile ommatidia and secondary lenses that scan the image created by stationary optics at the body surface. Decapod crustaceans, such as lobsters and crabs, can move their stalked eyes in drifts, tremors, and saccades independently of head and body movements.

Recording Eye Movements

Several methods are used to measure eye movements in humans and laboratory animals, some of great sensitivity and precision. The most commonly used clinical technique, electro-oculography, exploits a standing potential of about 6 mV that exists between the cornea and the back of the eye, the cornea being relatively positive (Figure 12.1). Electrodes placed around the eye will detect rotation of the globe as the positive pole swings one way and the negative pole the other. With this technique one can measure eye movements as small as $1-2°$ in amplitude. Another approach used in many human studies is to track the position of the pupillary border using infrared illumination and a suitable recording apparatus. This noninvasive technique can measure movements of less than a degree of arc.

Very small eye movements can be recorded by means of a contact lens bearing a small mirror: A light beam projected onto the mirror is reflected from it to a recording apparatus such as a camera or an array of photodetectors. As the eye moves, the angles of incidence and reflection of the light change, with the result that the light lever, as it is called, moves through twice the angle of the eye movement. The amplification achieved depends on the distance from the mirror to the recording apparatus, which can be very large. This method can resolve movements on the order of seconds of arc.

A recording method widely used in oculomotor research exploits the fact that a current is induced in a conductive wire exposed to an alternating magnetic field. In this technique, a coil of fine wire, the search coil, is attached directly to the eye or to a contact lens worn by the subject. When the subject's head is placed in an alternating magnetic field, the current induced in the search coil varies with eye position. The search-coil method provides a signal of eye position over a wide range and has a maximal sensitivity of about $0.25°$.

Positions and Motions of the Eyes

When a person directs the visual axes straight ahead, the eyes are said to be in primary position. Purely vertical or horizontal movements from primary position place the eyes in secondary positions. Tertiary positions are reached by movements from primary position combining vertical and horizontal components. Static misalignments of the visual axes are not uncommon and can interfere with fusion and depth perception. Strabismus or squint refers to misalignment when the observer attempts to fixate binocularly, either straight ahead or during movements of the eyes. If the eyes diverge, the condition is called exotropia, and if they converge,

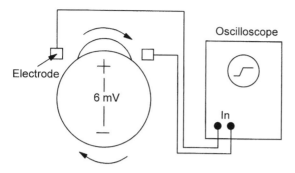

Figure 12.1. Method for recording the electro-oculogram (EOG).

esotropia. Exophoria and esophoria refer to misalignments that occur in the absence of fusional stimuli.

In vertebrates, the eye is suspended in the orbit by sets of muscles and is usually free to move in three dimensions. Rotations of the globe are conventionally described as occurring about three orthogonal axes (Figure 12.2A). Torsional movements take place about the visual axis, horizontal rotations about a vertical axis (dashed line in Figure 12.2A), and vertical rotations about a horizontal axis (dotted line in Figure 12.2A), all passing through some common point in the eye.

In animals with lateral eyes, such as fish, the direction of a horizontal movement of one eye is named for the part of the visual field toward which the visual axis is displaced. Thus, the eye is said to move nasally or temporally in the horizontal plane. Upward movements elevate the eye, and downward movements depress it. "Elevation" and "depression" also describe the corresponding movements in frontal-eyed animals, such as humans, but horizontal movements are named according to whether the visual axis is carried toward or away from the midline or nose. Movements toward the midline are called adduction (duction to) and movements away are called abduction (duction from). Torsional rotations about the visual axis are named for the direction in which the superior aspect of the eye moves. Intorsion rotates this point toward the nose, and extorsion rotates it away from the nose. These movements are illustrated in Figure 12.2B.

A separate set of terms is used to describe combined movements of the two eyes. These, too, refer to the directions in which the visual axes are displaced. Conjugate eye movements displace the visual axes of both eyes in the same direction, as if they were yoked together. Conjugate movements can be vertical, horizontal, and oblique. Vergence movements move the visual axes in opposite directions, either toward (convergence) or away (divergence) from each other.

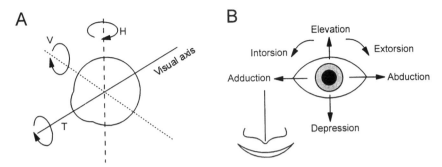

Figure 12.2. (A) Rotational axes of the eye. Horizontal rotations (H) occur about a vertical axis (dashed), and vertical rotations (V) about the horizontal axis (dotted), and torsional movements (T) about the visual axis. (B) Rotations of the human eye.

Muscles that Move the Eyes

In most vertebrates, each eye is moved by the activity of extraocular muscles that are attached to the bony orbit at one end and to the eyeball at the other. The geometry of the muscles and their attachments varies considerably among species. Four of the six extraocular muscles of humans are illustrated in Figure 12.3, which also shows the locations of the axes about which vertical and torsional movements are made. The axis for horizontal rotations is normal to the plane of the figure. The primary actions of the rectus muscles are easiest to see. The medial rectus adducts, the lateral abducts, the superior elevates, and the inferior (not shown) depresses the globe. The superior oblique passes through a small ring of bone, the trochlea, on the medial wall of the orbit, and acting around all three axes, it intorts, depresses, and abducts the eye. An inferior oblique muscle extends from the medial wall of the orbit and inserts on the underside of the eye. The lateral rectus is innervated by cranial nerve VI (the abducens nerve), and the superior oblique by cranial nerve IV (the trochlear nerve). The superior, inferior, and medial recti and the inferior oblique are innervated by cranial nerve III (the oculomotor nerve). Note that the term "oculomotor" sometimes refers specifically to cranial nerve III, and sometimes to all of the cranial nerves that innervate extraocular muscles.

Oculomotor Control Systems of the Brain Stem

The extraocular muscles must be precisely controlled to ensure proper alignment and coordinated movements of the two eyes. Because of the fine tolerances required by these functions, the nervous system has automated

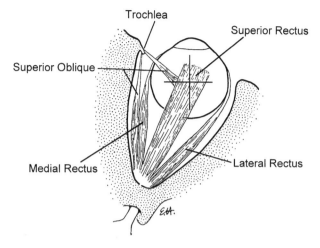

Figure 12.3. Geometry of extraocular muscles of the human right eye viewed from above. The eye is in primary position, i.e., the visual axis is directed straight ahead. The arms of the cross in the center of the eye represent the rotational axes of vertical and torsional movements. The vertical axis about which horizontal movements occur is normal to the page. The inferior rectus and inferior oblique muscles are not shown. (Adapted from F. H. Adler: *Gifford's Textbook of Ophthalmology*, 6th ed. Philadelphia: W. B. Saunders Co., 1957, with permission of the W. B. Saunders Company.)

them in subsystems that are under voluntary control, yet do not require one to think about how they are working. The difference between the oculomotor and somatic motor control systems can be appreciated from the degree to which they permit independent movements. For instance, one can wiggle one's right little finger at will, but one cannot voluntarily wiggle only one's right eye. Nor can humans move one eye up and the other eye down at the same time as chameleons and some fish can do.

An example of a low-level component of the coordinating circuitry is provided by the medial longitudinal fasciculus (MLF), a large myelinated tract of the brain stem. From the diagram of Figure 12.4 we see that a conjugate movement to the left requires that the lateral rectus of the left eye and the medial rectus of the right contract together, meaning that the left abducens (VI) nucleus and part of the right oculomotor (III) nucleus must be activated simultaneously. This synergism is accomplished through a special projection from the abducens nucleus on one side to the oculo-motor nucleus on the other (Figure 12.4). Internuclear neurons with their cell bodies in the abducens nucleus send their axons across the midline into the MLF. These ascend to the oculomotor nucleus and excite the

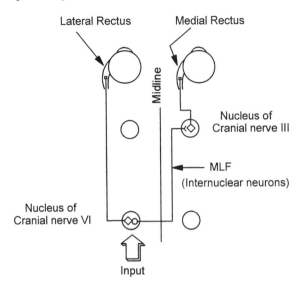

Figure 12.4. Connections of MLF involved in horizontal conjugate movement of the eyes.

motoneurons innervating the medial rectus. Thus, activation of the left abducens nucleus produces contraction of the left lateral rectus and, indirectly, the right medial rectus, resulting in a conjugate deviation to the left. All conjugate horizontal eye movements employ this circuitry.

Vertical and vergence eye movements require muscles innervated by the oculomotor and trochlear nerves, whose nuclei are located in the mesencephalon. It is not surprising, then, that the circuits that organize the premotor commands for vergence and vertical movements are also located in the mesencephalon and that lesions here interfere with vertical eye movements.

Quick and Slow Eye Movements

The oculomotor systems of vertebrate brains commonly generate two important subclasses of movements distinguished by their speed and designated by the unassuming terms quick and slow (Figure 12.5). These basic movements are incorporated into a variety of oculomotor programs. An example of a slow movement is smooth pursuit, in which the eyes track a moving target in a smooth, conjugate deviation. A person who is fixating an airplane passing high overhead is executing a smooth pursuit movement. Pursuit movements cannot ordinarily be performed voluntarily in

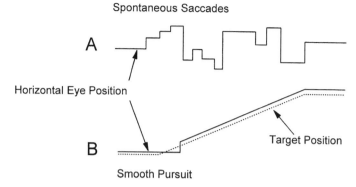

Figure 12.5. Quick and slow eye movements. (A) Schematic representation of saccadic eye movement of one eye. (B) Position of the eye as it pursues a target. Note the latency to pursuit onset and the initial saccade to fixate the stimulus. The horizontal axis is time.

the absence of a moving target. An example of a quick movement is the saccade, which is executed voluntarily during visual exploration and reading. A novel stimulus in the peripheral visual field may elicit a reflex saccade that brings the image of the stimulus to the fovea. This has been called the "visual grasp reflex." Conjugate movements may be slow (pursuit) or quick (saccades). Vergence movements are usually slow, but they may be assisted by quick conjugate movements of unequal size. The basic patterns occur in both voluntary and reflex eye movements.

There is considerable evidence that quick and slow eye movements are controlled by different brain systems. When a subject gets sleepy, quick movements disappear before slow movements. Administering a barbiturate, on the other hand, eliminates slow movements before suppressing saccades. Electrical stimulation of the superior colliculus evokes saccades, but not slow movements, whereas stimulation of the cerebellum can elicit slow movements alone.

Microscopic Eye Movements

When very sensitive measuring devices are used, such as the light-lever method described earlier, it is found that the human eye is never still. Even during intense voluntary fixation the eye continues to exhibit small drifts, a tremor, and periodic microsaccades. One can learn to suppress the microsaccades, but not the other two types of movements. This residual jitter of the eye is called physiologic nystagmus, and it is vital to visual function. When the position of the retinal image is decoupled from eye movement, as, for instance, by projecting the image directly on the retina with a tiny projector mounted on a contact lens, the stabilized image fades rapidly from perception. This is why we do not see the shadows cast by our retinal blood vessels unless we use some technique to cause these shadows to move on the retina.

Generation of Slow Eye Movements

The principal function of slow eye movements is to stabilize the retinal image (though not so perfectly as to cause the image to disappear from perception). Images are displaced on the retina either because objects move in the outside world or because the eye itself moves. Different reflex and voluntary mechanisms counteract the resulting image motion by matching eye rotation to stimulus movement. Image displacements due to head movements are opposed primarily by the vestibulo-ocular reflex. Large movements of the background evoke a smooth, following movement in the same direction, termed an optokinetic movement. If these slow movements evoked by vestibular or optokinetic stimulation are sufficiently large, a quick, anti-compensatory movement will drive the eye back toward the middle of the oculomotor range, and the slow movement will begin again. This combination of a slow movement and a quick movement is a form of nystagmus, which means a to-and-fro movement of the eyes (Figure 12.6). The slow movements of voluntary smooth pursuit have already been mentioned.

The Vestibulo-ocular Reflex

The vestibular apparatus located in the temporal bone of the skull has two components, the otolith organs and the semicircular canals. The otolith organs are sensitive to linear accelerations such as that due to gravity and that experienced when taking off in an airplane. Tilt of the head results in a signal from the otolith organs to the central nervous system that produces a partially compensatory torsion of the eyes. The most important signal in terms of oculomotor effects comes from the semicircular canals, which sense angular rotation of the head. During normal movements of the head, this signal represents the velocity with which the head is turning and produces a compensatory movement of the eyes in the opposite direction, the vestibulo-ocular reflex (VOR) (Figure 12.7). The gain of the VOR is the ratio of angular eye velocity to angular head velocity. Under many conditions this gain is close to 1, meaning that the reflex compensates nearly perfectly for the head rotation.

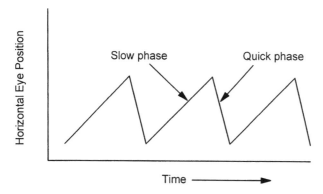

Figure 12.6. Nystagmus consisting of a slow movement followed by a quick resetting movement. Nystagmus can take other forms as well.

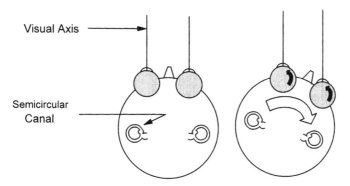

Figure 12.7. The VOR. Turning the head to the right activates the semicircular canals of the vestibular apparatus, which results in a conjugate, compensatory rotation of both eyes to the left, stabilizing the direction of gaze in space.

The circuitry responsible for the VOR is complex. The most direct pathway involves a three-neuron arc starting with the vestibular component of cranial nerve VIII. These axons synapse in the vestibular nuclei of the medulla, whose cells then project to the nuclei of VI and III. Less direct pathways involve other relays in the brain stem and a much longer one through the flocculus of the cerebellum and back to the brain stem.

A fascinating feature of the VOR is that its gain can be modified experimentally by having a subject wear special lenses that increase or decrease the degree of image displacement on the retina for a given rotation of the head. For instance, if the lenses move the image 2° for every degree of head rotation, the gain of the VOR is gradually reduced to about 0.5.

Similarly, if the image does not move far enough, the gain is increased. The gain of the reflex is modified automatically to maintain good stabilization of the retinal image during head rotation. The critical stimulus to adaptation seems to be motion of the retinal image when it is supposed to be stationary.

The cerebellum plays an important role in modifying the gain of the VOR. Destruction of the cerebellar flocculus eliminates the adaptive capacity or plasticity of the VOR, as it is sometimes called. The cerebellum receives all the information required to adjust the gain properly, because it is the target of both vestibular and visual projections. One function of VOR plasticity may be to compensate for physical changes in the brain that occur as an individual ages. The cerebellum has been characterized as a "repair shop" for the VOR, maintaining just the right conditions for optimal image stabilization during head rotation. A major focus of current research is to identify the locations within the cerebellum and/or brain stem where the plastic changes occur.

Optokinetic Movements

Displacements of the entire retinal image evoke slow eye movements that tend to oppose the displacement. A good example of this is so-called railroad nystagmus. When a person gazes from the window of a moving train, the eyes are irresistibly driven in the same direction as the rapidly passing telegraph poles or trees at the side of the track. After deviating to some angle, they return with a quick movement in the opposite direction; hence the term optokinetic nystagmus to describe the combined compensatory and anti-compensatory phases of the movement. The mechanisms responsible for optokinetic movements involve widely dispersed regions of the brain, including certain nuclei of the pretectum and even the visual cortex.

Optokinetic movements probably arise most often in response to movements of the head and body that displace the entire retinal image. Thus the mechanisms mediating optokinetic eye movements work synergistically with the VOR during natural body movements. The compensatory eye movements of these reflexes stabilize the retinal image of the background scenery, allowing the visual system to detect potentially significant movements of prey or predator against the stationary background.

Voluntary Smooth Pursuit or Tracking Movements

The initiation of smooth pursuit normally requires the presence of a moving visual stimulus. There is no smooth pursuit of auditory or somatic sensory stimuli, which the eye will attempt to fixate with saccades. The most important aspect of the stimulus for smooth pursuit is retinal slip (i.e., an actual movement of the image on the retina). Both the velocity and acceleration of retinal slip seem to be detected by the control system and to affect the eye movement. A second important parameter is position error, the static displacement of the image from the fovea. After-images created just off the fovea can generate smooth pursuit, although they may also elicit a sequence of saccades as the subject attempts in vain to move the image to the fovea.

Smooth pursuit allows the eye to stabilize the image of a moving target (e.g., an airplane) at the same time that the image of the background (e.g., the clouds) is moving on the retina. Thus, the control system has the complex task of stabilizing the image of the target while simultaneously disabling the optokinetic mechanisms that would normally oppose movement of the background image. Although pursuit requires a visual stimulus, it is evidently not controlled directly by the stimulus, because the eye continues to move even when the target disappears briefly (Figure 12.8). Also, eye velocity can momentarily exceed stimulus velocity, producing a slip in the opposite direction, without the movement stopping. A perfect match between eye velocity and stimulus velocity would stabilize the image on the fovea, eliminating retinal slip, but the eye moves none the less when the image is artificially stabilized for an instant. These observations indicate that the pursuit system uses a predictive strategy, generating an internal replica of target velocity and matching eye velocity to this over a certain period of time.

The pontine nuclei play a major role in smooth pursuit, relaying signals from cortical areas to the cerebellum. Following cerebellectomy there is total loss of smooth pursuit. The cerebellar region most clearly involved is the flocculus, where electrical stimulation elicits smooth conjugate movements and where neurons carry a signal of gaze velocity and eye velocity. Other cerebellar areas have also been implicated. Cells in the vestibular nuclei and nearby brain-stem structures discharge during pursuit and carry a signal proportional to eye velocity. These nuclei probably make up the final premotor substrate for pursuit.

Many cortical areas appear to be involved in smooth pursuit. Unilateral lesions in the striate cortex of monkeys irreversibly eliminate pursuit of objects in the "blind" hemifield, implying that subcortical systems alone cannot sustain this function. Lesions of area MT in the temporal lobe (see Figure 8.14) interfere with pursuit initiation in the area of visual field affected by the lesion. The posterior parietal cortex contains cells responding during smooth pursuit. Lesions of the frontal lobe, especially in area 8, the frontal eye fields (FEF), do not eliminate smooth pursuit, but de-

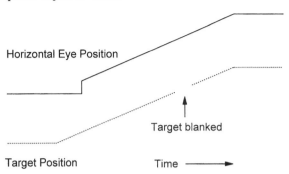

Horizontal Eye Position

Target blanked

Target Position   Time ───▶

Figure 12.8. Schematic illustration of predictive behavior during smooth pursuit. When the target disappears momentarily, the eye continues in the predicted direction of movement. To do this, the brain must have stored information about the past movement of the target, permitting it to estimate expected target position even when the target is not visible.

crease its effectiveness or gain (i.e., eye velocity/slip velocity). Lesions here eliminate the predictive capability of the system when animals track a repeated trajectory. The FEF contains cells that respond during smooth tracking, and electrical stimulation at some sites can evoked smooth movements. There is increased regional blood flow here during tracking.

In summary, several cerebral cortical areas are involved in the control of smooth pursuit, including striate cortex and superior temporal, parietal, and frontal areas. In the brain stem, the pons, cerebellum, and vestibular and neighboring nuclei form an important part of the premotor circuitry.

Generation of Saccadic Eye Movements

In contrast to slow eye movements, the principal function of quick eye movements is to displace the retinal image. Voluntary and reflex saccades are designed to move part of the image to a retinal area specialized for fine vision such as the fovea. To produce a saccade, the oculomotor neurons receive a burst of excitation to drive the eye swiftly to its new position and a new baseline level of firing to maintain the eye in that position (Figure 12.9). This burst-step pattern of input is generated by circuits in the paramedian pontine reticular formation for horizontal movements and in the rostral interstitial nucleus of the MLF of the midbrain for vertical movements. There exist connections between these areas to coordinate the horizontal and vertical components of oblique saccades.

A great deal of progress has been made in understanding the generation of saccadic eye movements by applying principles used by engineers in the

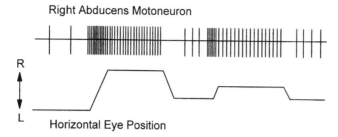

Figure 12.9. Schematic representation of the discharge of a motoneuron in the right abducens nucleus of a monkey as the animal makes saccades. There is a burst of activity before every rightward saccade, and the tonic level of discharge rises as the eye stops farther and farther to the right. The neuron goes silent during leftward saccades. This pattern of activity is organized automatically by neuronal circuitry of the brain stem.

analysis of control systems. To illustrate the basic strategy of this approach, it is necessary first to identify certain critical variables or quantities with which the system must deal. Saccadic eye movements are made in response to the appearance of a target of interest at some distance from the current point of fixation. The separation of the image of this stimulus from the fovea is called the retinal error of the stimulus, a quantity analogous to that of position error discussed earlier. The task of the oculomotor system is to create a saccadic eye movement equal to the retinal error in amplitude and direction. The oculomotor system could, in principle, use two strategies to do this. It could create a signal equal to retinal error and use this to drive the eye toward the target. Or it could combine the retinal-error signal and an internal signal of current eye position to create a signal of the target's position with respect to the head, and then issue a command to move the eye to the correct position in the orbit (Figure 12.10). Under most circumstances, the result would be the same, but the underlying strategies require very different computations by the oculomotor system.

The distinction between these two strategies was made clear in an experiment by D. L. Sparks and L. E. Mays, illustrated schematically in Figure 12.11: A monkey was trained to make saccades to a target (asterisk) that appeared briefly right above the fixation point (F) and then disappeared. Before the eye could move upward to where the target appeared, the eye was driven to a new position by electrical stimulation of the superior colliculus. The retinal-error signal (e_r) was purely vertical, and if this were translated directly into a movement vector, the result would be a vertical saccade. However, if the control system computed the actual position of the target with respect to the head (T_h) and positioned the eye

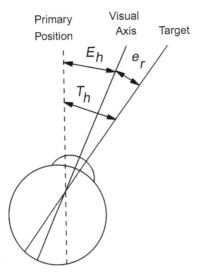

Figure 12.10. Critical angles defining target location. The eye is deviated by angle E_h (eye in the head) from the primary position. The target's image is displaced by angle e_r (retinal error) from the fovea. The sum of e_r and E_h is the target's position with respect to the head, T_h.

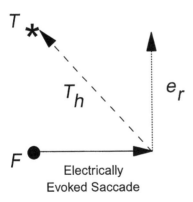

Figure 12.11. Schematic representation of an experiment showing that the saccadic control system can compute target position with respect to the head. The alert monkey fixates the point F. A target (asterisk) is flashed briefly directly above the fixation point and disappears. Before the eye can move to the target, the eye is displaced laterally by electrical stimulation of the superior colliculus, so that the eye must now move to the original target from a new starting position. The retinal-error information (e_r) would specify a purely vertical saccade, whereas an oblique saccade would occur if the saccadic system had computed target position with respect to the head (T_h).

accordingly, the saccade would be oblique. The saccades in fact were oblique, indicating that the system generated a signal corresponding to target position, not retinal error. This implies a computational complexity in the circuits responsible for saccade generation that has a parallel in the predictive character of smooth pursuit described earlier.

Several formal models of the saccadic control system can account for this kind of behavior. The strategy in using these models is to identify the operations required to carry out a function and then search out the neural structures that appear to perform these operations. As a first step, the system is conceptualized as a network of boxes, each performing some elemental function of the overall operation. The boxes are interconnected in such a way as to realize the desired behavior. Quantitative predictions from these models can be compared to the actual performance of the oculomotor system. A good match suggests that the assumptions of the model may be correct and that one should look for neural circuitry capable of performing the theoretical operations. The experimenter seeks an isomorphism (an identity of form) between the functional architecture of the nervous system and the functional architecture of the model.

Most current theories of saccade control are based on a seminal model proposed by D. A. Robinson that, although extensively modified and elaborated in recent years, will serve to illustrate the approach (Figure 12.12). In this model, the oculomotor system computes target direction with respect to the head and drives the eye until the visual axis has the same direction as the target. The model assumes that there exists within the circuits of the brain stem a signal E_h proportional to current eye position in the head. This is a reasonable assumption, because the oculomotor neurons require such a signal to maintain the eye in its current position (Figure 12.9). When this signal is combined with that for retinal error (e_r), the sum is equivalent to the position or direction of the target with respect to the head $(T_h$ in Figure 12.10). After a certain delay, this signal is fed to a mechanism that subtracts current eye position (E_h) from target position to produce a signal of motor error (e_m), which is the immediate input to the saccade-generating machinery of the brain stem. When a saccade is triggered, the eye movement causes E_h to change in the direction of T_h, and movement continues until these two signals are equal. At that point e_m goes to zero and the eye stops. The delay mechanism is required to prevent the signal T_h from changing at the right-hand summing point during the brief instant that the saccade is occurring and E_h is changing.

The Robinson model has been modified and extended in recent years to accommodate many complexities associated with the control of gaze. For instance, gaze direction can be changed by both head and eye move-

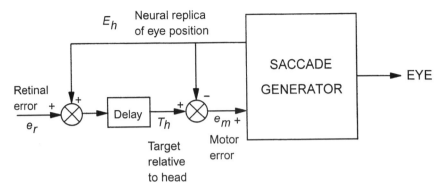

Figure 12.12. Schematic representation of local feedback control by the saccadic system.

ments, so there must be important interactions between the oculomotor mechanisms and the vestibular system. Also, saccades of different sizes can be controlled in different ways, and gaze shifts of comparable amplitudes can be accomplished by varying combinations of head and eye movements. Analysis of the circuitry underlying these phenomena remains an active area of research.

Higher-Level Systems Controlling Saccadic Eye Movements

Many cortical areas appear to be involved in the targeting and guidance of saccades. Electrical stimulation of visual cortex evokes saccades, and lesions here impair or eliminate visually guided saccades. Electrical activation of the frontal eye fields causes conjugate saccades to the opposite side, and cells in this area discharge prior to saccades to visual targets, but not before "spontaneous" saccades. The frontal eye fields were long thought to be the cortical "motor areas" for voluntary eye movements, but this analogy with the primary motor cortex is not helpful and has largely been abandoned. Recent studies have found neurons in the parietal lobe that discharge prior to eye movements.

The visual cortex, the frontal eye fields, and the parietal lobe all project to subcortical targets involved in saccadic eye movements. One of these is the superior colliculus of the midbrain, which also receives a direct retinal input (see Figure 4.8). The superior colliculus is involved in reflex orientation to novel stimuli and probably in other visually guided behaviors as well. Its destruction in non-primate mammals results in severe deficits in visual orienting responses. Primates suffer less impairment following permanent collicular lesions, but marked deficits can be demonstrated by focal injection of local anesthetics while the animal is performing an oculomotor task. Neurons in the deeper collicular layers discharge prior to voluntary saccadic eye movements, and some of these cells project to the brain-stem regions that provide premotor input to the oculomotor neurons. Focal electrical stimulation of the colliculus produces saccades whose direction and amplitude are related to the retinotopic sensory coordinates at the stimulus site. The saccade will leave the visual axis pointing at the receptive fields of cells recorded at the site prior to stimulation. Thus, the superior colliculus appears to contain a motor map of saccade vectors that is, in part at least, in spatial register with the retinotopic sensory map.

Experimental observations on cells of the superior colliculus support the notion that motor commands guiding saccades involve an ensemble or distributed code. Many cells in the superior colliculus have large visual receptive fields, and cells in the deeper layers have large movement fields; that is, they discharge before saccades to a number of locations in visual space. Thus, the discharge of any given cell is ambiguous with respect to the location of a stimulus or a saccade target. As discussed in Chapter 9 with respect to retinal and cortical cells, the large visual receptive fields of collicular neurons indicate that the point image among such cells is large. Similarly, the large movement fields imply that premotor activity occurs in a large patch of output cells before saccades to a given point in visual space. The position of the active population varies systematically and retinotopically with the location of the stimulus and the movement vector of the resulting saccade. How, then, might the stimulus point or saccade target be represented in the large area of cell discharge?

The effects of electrical stimulation in different parts of the colliculus suggest that retinotopically organized connectional gradients link the colliculus functionally to the premotor circuitry responsible for saccade generation. Putting this together with the large, retinotopically organized point image led to the model of Figure 12.13, in which the active region (understood in either a sensory or motor context) serves to assemble the saccadic command by its intersection with the connectional gradients. As the stimulus or saccade target moves around in visual space, the zone of activity moves around in the colliculus, changing the composition of the output signal appropriately. Spatial information is not lost in the large receptive fields or movement fields, but is encoded in motor coordinates. Alternative models of collicular coding have been advanced to address findings not explained by the simple system of Figure 12.13, but all of these have in common that points in the visual field and saccade targets are represented by neural activity in large populations of collicular neurons.

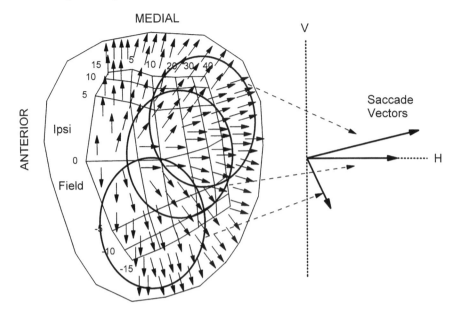

Figure 12.13. Hypothetical means of encoding saccade direction and amplitude by ensembles of neurons in the superior colliculus. The small arrows symbolize the movement components or "minivectors" contributed by neural discharge at a particular site. These are shown superimposed on the sensory retinotopic map. The oval profiles represent the locations of activity prior to three saccades whose directions and amplitudes are indicated by the large arrows in the diagram at right; V, vertical; H, horizontal. The superior colliculus diagrammed here is that of the cat, which has a rostral representation of the ipsilateral visual field. (Reprinted, with permission, from J. McIlwain: Distributed spatial coding in the superior colliculus: a review. *Visual Neuroscience* 6:3–13, 1991.)

Further Reading

Büttner-Ennever, J. A. (ed.) (1988). *Reviews of Oculomotor Research. Vol. 3: Neuroanatomy of the Oculomotor System.* Amsterdam: Elsevier.

Carpenter, R. H. S. (1977). *Movements of the Eyes.* London: Pion.

Fuchs, A. F., Kanecko, C. R. S., and Scudder, C. A. (1985). Brainstem control of saccadic eye movements. *Annual Review of Neuroscience* 8:307–37.

Land, M. H. (1981). Optics and vision in invertebrates. In *Handbook of Sensory Physiology*, vol. 7, part 6B, ed. H. Autrum, pp. 471–592. Berlin: Springer-Verlag.

Lisberger, S. G., Morris, E. J., and Tychsen, L. (1987). Visual motion processing and sensory-motor integration for smooth pursuit eye movements. *Annual Review of Neuroscience* 10:97–129.

McIlwain, J. T. (1991). Distributed spatial coding in the superior colliculus: a review. *Visual Neuroscience* 6:3–13.

Miles, F. A., and Lisberger, S. G. (1981). Plasticity in the vestibulo-ocular reflex: a new hypothesis. *Annual Review of Neuroscience* 4:273–99.

Robinson, D. A. (1975). Oculomotor control signals. In *Basic Mechanisms of Ocular Motility and Their Clinical Implications*, ed. G. Lennerstrand and P. Bach-y-Rita, pp. 337–74. Oxford: Pergamon.

Sparks, D. L., and Mays, L. E. (1983). The spatial localization of saccade targets. I. Compensation for stimulation-induced perturbations in eye position. *Journal of Neurophysiology* 49:45–63.

Wehner, R. (1981). Spatial vision in arthropods. In *Handbook of Sensory Physiology*, vol. 7, part 6C, ed. H. Autrum, pp. 285–616. Berlin: Springer-Verlag.

Wurtz, R. H., and Goldberg, M. E. (eds.) (1989). *The Neurobiology of Saccadic Eye Movements*. Amsterdam: Elsevier.

INDEX

Made in the USA
Lexington, KY
09 August 2013